First One Home

First One to Survive

BY
Barbara Lopez with
LCpl. Josef Lopez

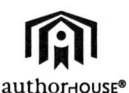
authorHOUSE

AuthorHouse™
1663 Liberty Drive
Bloomington, IN 47403
www.authorhouse.com
Phone: 1-800-839-8640

© 2009 Barbara Lopez with LCpl. Josef Lopez. All rights reserved.

No part of this book may be reproduced, stored in a retrieval system, or transmitted by any means without the written permission of the author.

First published by AuthorHouse 10/7/2009

ISBN: 978-1-4490-1260-1 (e)
ISBN: 978-1-4490-1266-3 (sc)
ISBN: 978-1-4490-1265-6 (hc)

Printed in the United States of America
Bloomington, Indiana

This book is printed on acid-free paper.

Table of Contents

Preface		ix
January 2006	The News	1
Sunday, October 1	The Call	4
Sunday, October 1	The Long Wait	6
Monday, October 2	The Search	9
Tuesday, October 3	Getting Ready	12
Wednesday, October 4	The Flight	17
Thursday, October 5	Germany	28
Friday, October 6	The Flight to Bethesda	38
Saturday, October 7	First Day of Treatment	46
Sunday, October 8	Near Death	53
Monday, October 9	Columbus Day	60
Tuesday, October 10	Hospital Gets Back to Normal	63
Wednesday, October 11	Movie Day	72
Thursday, October 12	Coming off the Ventilator	76
Friday, October 13	Glen's Visit	83
Saturday, October 14	Sitting up and Getting a Shave	85
Sunday, October 15	Steven's Birthday and His Last Day	88
Monday, October 16	I Am Alone	91
Tuesday, October 17	Out of ICU!!	96
Wednesday, October 18	Settling in on the Fifth Floor	100
Thursday, October 19	Out of Room & Confrontation with Doctor	103
Friday, October 20	IVIG Treatment & Roommate Drama	107
Saturday, October 21	Confrontation with Nurse	110
Sunday, October 22	Visitors and Phone Calls	116

Monday, October 23	Haircut	131
Tuesday, October 24	Shave	136
Wednesday, October 25	Lots of Visitors	141
Thursday, October 26	More Visitors	143
Friday Morning, October 27	Brian's Surgery & More Visitors	146
Friday Afternoon, October 27	Brian's Meltdown	150
Saturday, October 28	Things Quiet Down	159
Sunday, October 29	Marine Corps Marathon & Lou's Escape	165
Monday, October 30	Long Distance Arrangements	171
Tuesday, October 31	Halloween	175
Brendon's Story		178
Halloween Night		180
Wednesday, November 1 to Sunday, November 5	One Month	183
Monday, November 6 and Tuesday, November 7	Feeling Bad	185
Wednesday, November 8	Marine Corps Birthday Party	188
Thursday, November 9	IVIG Treatment	191
Friday, November 10	Marine Corps Birthday	194
Saturday, November 11	Taking Joe to the Navy Lodge	197
Sunday, November 12	Relaxing Day	200
Monday, November 13	Acinebactor	203
Tuesday, November 14	Our Last Day?	206
Wednesday, November 15	Leaving Bethesda	209
November 16 thru December 3	Rehab	214
Monday, December 4	Lou's Funeral	219

December 8	Joe Comes Home!	221
Ups and Downs		223
Ambulance and Re-admittance to the Hospital		228
April 21	Marine Parents Conference	230
April 23 to 27	Preparing for Homecoming	233
April 28	Homecoming!!	234
Smallpox Vaccination Facts		238
Postscript		251
Acknowledgments		257

Preface

Shortly after my son, Josef, was deployed to Iraq, he developed a strange numbness in his legs. I began keeping a journal to keep track of his symptoms, and later his recovery. I also used the journal to monitor my husband's illness, and ultimate death. Later, as a form of therapy for myself, I began to write my story from the notes in my journal.

Within days, we knew that Joe's illness was extremely rare and often fatal. It is so rare that most of the doctors we have met have never heard of it. One doctor, who knew how lethal ADEM can be, gasped and exclaimed "I'm amazed that you survived!" Joe's official diagnosis was Acute Disseminated Encephalomyelitis (ADEM), triggered by the smallpox vaccination he was given just days before deployment. The military reinstated the smallpox vaccination program in 2002 and Joe is only the fourth person to develop ADEM from it, and the first to have long-term survival.

As time passed, and we met others with adverse reactions to military vaccinations, the idea of writing a book began to gel. We began to question why our military gives such a dangerous vaccination for a disease that hasn't been seen, anywhere in the world, for more than 30 years. Why do we vaccinate for a disease that the World Health Organization declared as "eradicated" in 1980? We have found young people with many types of adverse reactions, who must now deal with life-threatening and life long illnesses. Many are being discharged or medically retired, instead of living out their dreams of a military career. In the current economic climate, we question the expenses to the taxpayers for, not only the smallpox program, but the expenses the taxpayers must bear for these unfortunate few, for the rest of their lives.

In writing this book, we speak for all the young Marines, Soldiers, and Airmen who have had their lives turned upside down by a shot, or shots, meant to protect them. We speak for them as we ask why these vaccinations are given, and how they can be made safer.

I also wrote this book as a beacon of hope for those who are challenged by rare diseases. Joe has proven that you must be a fighter, never giving up, always striving for the next level of success. From those first days in ICU, when he spent hours trying to get his hands to respond to give a "thumbs up"; I knew that he would fight his hardest. When they said he might never stand on his own, he worked till he could. When they said he might never walk, he worked till he could. He may need frequent rest stops, but he walks. He also races, even in marathons, with a special made hand cycle.

Our message to all who read this book is this: educate yourself, be aware of dangers and if the worst happens, be pro-active and insist on the best treatment available. Fight hard, and never give up, you just might be the one to break all the records. Be a fighter and be a survivor.

Chapter 1

January 2006

The News

It was a cold, snowy day when we got the news. I knew was coming, it was only a matter of time, but I was dreading it just the same. My 19 year old son brought the news to us at the end of his "drill weekend" with his Marine reserve unit. He was going to Iraq, and that was that. It was bound to happen but I can't say that I was pleased.

For my husband, Joe's dad, it took a few days for the news to sink in. Lou was sinking deeper and deeper into the brain fog that Alzheimer's disease brings. The diagnosis had been made about a year earlier, but we had suspected it for several years. He had already been through the early and middle stage drugs, and we knew that he was entering the final stages. I explained to him over and over again that Joe would be going away soon and his reaction was different each time. One time he would be overjoyed that Joe was going to be traveling (as if he were leaving on vacation), another time he would worry that he could be injured, but most of the time he was too confused to understand at all.

I had always been a worrier, so that's what I did. I worried about Lou sinking into the abyss of Alzheimer's, I worried about Joe going off to war, and I worried about my other son who lived much too far away. I worried about what I would do if Lou didn't make it until Joe's homecoming. Should tell him if his dad passed away while he was in Iraq? I finally asked Joe about it and we decided that I would not — he would need to keep his mind on the task at hand.

I wanted to be as informed as possible, so I joined the Key Volunteer network, a group of Marine wives and mothers who helped relay information between the Corps and the families of deployed Marines. By becoming a Key Volunteer, I would hear the news first, then pass it on to the families in my group.

Joe left for training, first to Ohio, then to California. He trained for several months, during the summer, in the middle of the desert. It was actually hotter in the California desert than it was in Iraq and, finally, after four months, they were ready. They were allowed a quick trip home before returning for the final days of packing gear for the trip. When I saw him, I was amazed at how lean and muscular he was. He was obviously in top physical shape.

We had just one short week with him then, all too soon, it was time to take him to the airport for his trip back to California. As he told his father goodbye, Lou said "have a great trip. I sure wish I was going with you. You're going to love Europe." He was oblivious to the truth, sinking deep into his disease and Joe was convinced that it was the last time he would see his father alive. I worried about him going off to war with that thought, but I couldn't do anything to change it.

I watched him as he went through the security checkpoint, then he turned and waved as he moved up the escalator toward the gate. I had always hated saying good bye, always cried at airports, and I was crying again as I exited the door to the parking lot. As I walked toward the street, I looked down at the ground and spotted a lone penny lying near the curb. "A lucky penny," I thought, "perhaps this is a sign," and bent down to pick it up. As I sat in my car and watched the airplane gracefully climb into the sky and turn toward the west, I was optimistic. I had to believe that, no matter what happened, everything would turn out alright. I had to believe that, somehow, everything would work out. I could never have guessed the truth but through it all, this belief would sustain me. And the signs would keep coming.

Chapter 2

Sunday, October 1

The Call

My journey started with a phone call, that terrible phone call that all parents dread … the phone call they hope they will never get. The one where your child is on the other line saying, "Mom, I'm in the hospital". But in my case, it was so much worse……my child was on the other side of the world…..and in a war zone. Yes, it all started with that phone call.

I hadn't had a good night's sleep for over a week, ever since that other terrible phone call — the one where he told me they were leaving the United States the next day. When the phone rang at 4:00 am, I didn't answer it fast enough and it went to voice mail. "Hi, mom, it's me, it must be early there, and you're probably still asleep. I'll try to call again in a couple of hours. I'm in the hospital but it's not real bad. I'll call later. Bye." What? In the hospital? What could have happened? Gunshot, explosion, vehicle accident? My mind raced, but I never could have guessed the truth. I tried to sleep, with the phone right next to me, but sleep didn't come.

The second call came about three hours later, the ringing startled me, even though I was waiting and wishing for it to happen. Hello (please let it be him), and there he was! "Hi, mom, it's me." What's happening? "I'm in the hospital in Iraq, but the good news is that the doctors think they know what it is and how to treat it." He proceeded to tell me how his legs had started to go numb, and how the numbness grew worse and spread upward until he couldn't stand. He said the doctors suspected a virus and might transfer him to a hospital in Germany. He chuckled when he told me that the highlight of his day had been when they put in the catheter. I chuckled too, imagining my strong Marine, who had never had a major illness in his life, being told that he was about to get a catheter inserted! I questioned his treatment — just Tylenol for the headache. Nothing else hurt; but he couldn't feel his legs, just numbness from the waist down…. I thought for a minute of my own numbness from the waist down, during the C-section I had on the day he was born….

Then, as if to reassure me, he mentioned the ventilator that was sitting beside his bed "just in case the numbness moves up to my lungs". What? What had he just said? Now my mind was really racing, how bad could this be? How bad could it get? I heard a female voice, and then he said he had to go. No, wait, not yet, what about the ventilator? "Don't worry," he said, "the doctors here know what they are doing". No, wait, can you call me later, before you go to sleep tonight? He asked the nurse then relayed her answer. "She says she'll bring the satellite phone back in a couple of hours so I can call you again." Well, OK, take care of yourself, don't forget to call, I'll keep the phone with me. "OK, don't worry." OK, love ya. Then he was gone, and that was the last I heard from him.

Chapter 3

Sunday, October 1

The Long Wait

Now, if that call had come from a local hospital, I would have been in the car and headed toward the Emergency Room in no time flat. But what do you do when the call is from the other side of the world? You do the only thing you CAN do — you wait for the next call. It was Sunday morning and my husband was still asleep, as he moved deeper into the Alzheimer's disease, sleep was a blessing. I didn't want to wake him. I didn't think he could comprehend it. There would be no more sleep for me, so I quietly got dressed, did a little house cleaning, and sent some e-mails.

Lisa was my Key Volunteer Coordinator and also the wife of Joe's commanding officer, and I sent the first e-mail to her. The second e-mail went to my Aunt Velda, who lives in northern California. She knows lots of people, is very good at the computer and good at finding out stuff. I called Major Corrado, the Family Readiness Officer for Joe's unit in Kansas City; he was not aware of the situation but agreed to contact his superiors. I got the impression that he thought I was a hysterical mother, which was OK, as long as he was willing to search for information.

I went outside to mow the lawn but kept the cell phone on me the entire time. I come from a large and confusing family. My parents divorced when I was young, then both remarried, so I have full, half and step siblings. I called my sister, Teri, and had her call my mother's side of the family. Then I called my dad & step mother, and was glad when Grace answered the phone. I broke down as I told her the story and asked her to tell my dad, and to call my other son, Steven, who lived in Albuquerque. How do you tell your child that his only brother may be dying?

I went back to the lawn, finishing the front and moving to the back yard. Soon my phone rang, but it wasn't Joe, it was Steven. He had gotten the phone call from his grandma, but it had gone to his voicemail and he hadn't been able to get her when he called back. So he called me to see what was wrong, and I was devastated to have to tell him! I knew he would be sitting by the phone worrying until we heard from Joe again.

I went back to the lawn, glad to have something physical to do to keep myself busy. Soon, Lou appeared at the back door. I shut the mower off and went in the house to tell him the news. He didn't fully understand, and was happy that Joe might be coming home. "Maybe in a box," I thought. I had some Kava Kava, herbs known to calm nerves, so I took a couple. As the day wore on, I took it several more times. They seemed to help and I thought they were better for me than a prescription medication. I was calmer and able to think more clearly.

The phone rang again, it was my Aunt Velda from California and she had been doing some research. "This sounds like Guillien-Barre", she said, "and if it is, you better start making plans to go to him. He may not make it home". Well, that was comforting — but it got me to thinking, and I called Steven in Albuquerque again. I knew that Lou was not well enough to travel and, if I had to go, I didn't want to go alone. Steven agreed to go with me and said he'd start making arrangements with his employer. I called my friend, Julie, who is a nurse married to a physician's assistant and they both agreed that Joe's symptoms sounded like Guillien-Barre.

It was mid afternoon, so I ate some lunch and waited for a phone call. Iraq was nine hours ahead of our time and I knew it must be getting close to bedtime for the patients. The call could come at any time.

By 3:00 pm, midnight in Iraq, I knew something had gone terribly wrong. I had to start getting ready for work; the 5 pm to 9 pm shift at Taco Bueno. It was a new job for me, the restaurant had only been open a couple of weeks and I worked as a cashier in the evenings. It was my second job, and I worked there to pay off the credit card bills that my husband had secretly charged up. I had learned, too late, that many Alzheimer's patients do this as their financial common sense leaves them. Since he was home during the day (while I was at my main job), it was easy for him get the mail and hide the bills from me. By the time I discovered what he'd done, there were thousands of dollars of debt. I had worked two, and sometimes, three jobs at a time for over a year to pay down the debt.

Before I left for work, I left a note with my work phone number on it and instructed Lou to call me immediately if he got any calls — especially one from Joe. He said he would, but I wasn't sure that he would remember. I spent the night questioning every call that came in to the restaurant, but none were for me. When I got home, Lou confirmed that nobody had called. I tried to call Major Corrado but got his answering machine.

Chapter 4

Monday, October 2

The Search

I kept the silent phone by my bed, and tossed and turned all night. I worked as a secretary in a high school counseling center and it was an especially busy time of year for me. School had just begun and I was still enrolling new students, while helping returning students settle into the proper classes for the year. I had lots of work to do, and taking a day off was just not possible. Besides, I thought I could get more done at work than I could at home — with Lou asking the same questions, over and over again. So, I gathered up my collection of phone numbers and headed out the door. One of the first things I did was send an e-mail to the entire staff, asking them for advice. I knew that my co-workers had a variety of different lifestyles, contacts, and knowledge and I knew I would get some good advice from them. I also started calling and e-mailing everyone I could think of who could help me. When you need information quickly, your network of friends and acquaintances are VERY valuable.

As the day wore on, I got lots of good advice: call the Red Cross, call your congressman, call the Marine Corps., etc. I tried everything. Lisa e-mailed that she had heard from her husband in Iraq but all he knew was that Joe had been airlifted to Balad on Saturday. My congressman's office said they'd check into it and call me back. I sent an e-mail to MarineParents.com. My friend, Doris, called her husband (a doctor) and he also suspected Guillain-Barre syndrome. The local Red Cross had been constructing a new building and was in the process of moving into their new offices on that very day, but I talked to a extremely helpful lady named Pat. She didn't even know where her phone was (she was using someone else's), but agreed to see what she could do. I called the Marines again, still no word.

It was late afternoon when Pat, from the Red Cross, called me back. School was out and almost everyone had gone home, and Pat had finally found him. My heart raced as she told me what she knew. My Joe was in a hospital in Balad, Iraq but was in a coma and on a ventilator. I knew it. I just knew it. She said that they planned to transfer him to Germany that night (it was already after midnight in Iraq) and I should hear from the doctor sometime tomorrow. Well, at least I knew.

I started walking toward the main office, but two of my co-workers stopped me. They could see the pain in my face. I got out the words, "He's not breathing on his own" before breaking down and we stood in the hall, embracing and crying together. They both agreed that I should go to him as soon as possible. Our principal walked out of his office, headed for home, and stopped to hear the news. His only words to me were "I want you on the first plane you can get on, we'll take care of things here". I knew then, that my job would be OK, one less thing for me to worry about. Before leaving school, I called my employer at Taco Bueno and got the same response, "Do what you have to do and your job will be waiting when you return."

When I got home, I tried to explain it all to Lou, but he still didn't understand how serious Joe's condition was. I called Steven to tell him to be ready and learned that he had already talked to his employer and everything was set on his end. I also called the rest of the family, then settled in for another restless night, waiting for a call from Germany.

I had seen something on TV about the medivac flights from Iraq, and I knew that they left late at night, with the runway lights dimmed and the airplane lights off so they wouldn't be shot down. I knew it was dangerous, and I knew that Joe would be unconscious and breathing with the aide of a ventilator. It was hard to sleep.

Chapter 5

Tuesday, October 3

Getting Ready

Once again, the phone woke me up in the wee hours of the morning — 5:00 a.m. this time. I grabbed it quickly, but it had already gone to voice mail. How many times had it rang? Twice? Three times? I wasn't sure. I waited for the voice mail tone. Ding-dong. There it was. I grabbed the phone and pressed the buttons. The message was from a doctor in Germany — Joe's doctor — he had just examined him and wanted me to call him back. He left his phone number, but my cell phone didn't seem to be able to call it.

I no longer had a "land line" phone; I had it taken out about a year earlier when I discovered that many of the purchases Lou had made were from telephone telemarketers. Since I couldn't stop him from buying (taking the cards away didn't help as they already had the card numbers), I finally had the phone taken out. All I had was the cell phone which I left with Lou each day while I was at work. He had a phone to use, but the telemarketers didn't have the number. I called my cell phone company and I was told that I didn't have international calling on my phone, but I could add it during normal working hours. I didn't want to wait to talk to the doctor, so who could help me?

I thought of my friend, Patty, who had been stationed in Germany when she was in the Air Force, and now lived in Kansas City. Surely Patty would know what to do. I called her and found that she was awake and getting her kids ready to go to school. She agreed to call the doctor for me and have him call me back. Patty is a true friend.

Soon, my phone rang again and it was Dr. Marco, the doctor from Germany. He gave me the news. He had examined Joe, done a lumbar puncture and an MRI, and found lesions in the brain and spinal cord. Joe had stopped breathing and was on a ventilator and they had put him into a medically induced coma to keep him calm. He was only responding to great pain, his condition was Very Serious, and his diagnosis was transverse myelitis. The next hospital plane would be on Friday and Joe could be on it if his medical condition stabilized. Dr. Marco thought it would be a good idea for a couple of family members to travel to Germany to try to get a response from Joe, as that would greatly improve his chances of surviving the flight home. He told me that because his condition was listed as Very Serious (the worst category), the military would pay for up to 3 family member's travel. I told him that Steven and I would like to come and he agreed to get the paperwork started. He told me someone would be calling me in a few hours and I gave him my work phone number. I made phone calls to Patty, thanking her for making the call to Germany, and to Steven, telling him to get ready to go. Then I got dressed and went to work.

I didn't know how long I'd be gone, so I arranged for a substitute for the rest of the week. Looking back, I was SO naïve! I spent the day arranging my desk and leaving detailed instructions for Angie, my sub. Neither of us realized that it would be a very long term assignment for her. When Shelia (our head secretary) told me that I had 82 days of sick leave that I could use, I laughed and said, "I sure hope I don't need it all"! But I went to the school administrative offices and filled out a Family Medical Leave Form, just in case. On my way back, I found a penny on the ground, a lucky penny. Was it a sign? It made me smile and gave me encouragement.

I called Lou's doctor, who said that he needed as much stability as possible. If there was nobody to come to our home and stay with him, he needed to be with someone he knew. I called different members of the family and was thrilled when my sister, Teri, offered to let Lou stay with her while I was gone. He wasn't interested, insisting that he could spend a few days at home alone but, after I threatened to find a nursing home for him, he finally agreed to go to Teri's house. He'd always been stubborn, but I knew that I couldn't leave him alone. It was one argument I just had to win.

I started getting calls from Sgt. Nichols, my Marine liaison, as he arranged for travel for Steven and me. I called Taco Bueno and told them to write me out of the schedule until further notice. When I called Major Corrado, in Kansas City, and told him what I knew, his demeanor changed and he no longer talked like he thought I was being hysterical. I sent e-mails to everyone I could think of, asking them to pray for Joe. At the end of the day, Shelia & Debbie (our financial secretary) came to me with an envelope full of money that the staff had donated so I would have one less thing to worry about. It brought me to tears once again; friends don't get any better than that.

When I got home from work, I spotted my neighbor, Jerry, in his yard across the street. I told him what was happening and he agreed to watch the house and collect the mail while I was gone. Then I went in to face Lou. He wasn't happy, wanted to argue about why he couldn't go to Germany with me, where he was going to stay, etc. But he finally saw that I wasn't going to back down and agreed to go to Teri's house — but only for a few days. OK, I was happy to get that much and went in to pack. Having never been to Europe, I decided to take jeans & t-shirts (for comfort) and a sweater in case it was cold. I also packed a bag for the airplane, things to read, bills that needed to be paid, a notebook, vitamins, even a snack. Lou packed his own bag; he always packed twice as many clothes as he needed, so I didn't need to help him with it. I got his prescriptions together and made a list for Teri, so she could sort them out for him every day. I had to stop by Wal-Mart then went to Taco Bueno for burritos and cheesecake chimichangas to eat on the drive. Lou loved the chimichangas and I knew that they would calm him down. It was nearly 9:00 when we finally left town.

It was a 3-½ hour drive from my house to Teri's house, just south of Tulsa, and that night it seemed to take twice as long. The miles drug on and on, Lou was nervous and talked constantly. As is the case with Alzheimer's patients, he talked about the same things over and over again. I tried turning on the radio but he would turn it down so he could talk to me. I tried talking about the weather, the traffic, the trees, the towns we were going past. Nothing worked; he would start repeating what he had just told me as soon as I stopped to take a breath. The only time he was quiet was when my cell phone rang, and I talked to my pastor. I asked him to pray for Joe and he promised to call again in a few days. It was around midnight when we finally got to Teri's house; she had left the front door open so we unpacked the car and let ourselves in. Lou went to bed, he was exhausted, and I jumped in the shower. I got to sleep somewhere around 1 a.m., but woke up several times to check the clock. I was so afraid that I'd miss my flight the next morning.

Meanwhile, in Albuquerque, Steven had also been talking to Sgt. Nichols and made arrangements for a 6 am flight. He gave his boss the news, then spent the evening washing clothes and packing for the trip.

Chapter 6

Wednesday, October 4

The Flight

My alarm woke me up at 3:45 am and I quietly got ready to leave. I didn't want to wake Lou and get him started talking again. Teri had left some cereal out for me and I was careful to make as little noise as possible. At 4:20, I went to unlock the front door for my other sister, Sheri, and was surprised to see her standing on the porch. What timing. We put my things in her car and headed toward the airport. It was good to have her to talk to, we had a nice conversation and it calmed my nerves. Sheri and Teri are identical twins, but their personalities are as different as night and day. I was 12 years old when they were born, but even with the age difference, we have always been close. I could talk to them about anything, and even when they weren't getting along with each other, they always got along with me. Sheri dropped me off at the United Airlines entrance at 5:00 a.m., we said our goodbyes and she went on to work. I checked my bags, went through security and found my gate. While I was waiting, I decided to check on Joe's condition.

Since my cell phone wouldn't call overseas, the Marine Corps had given me a special phone number to call where I could be patched through. When I called that number, I talked to Donna who told me not to get on the plane. She said that Joe might be moved later that day, not Friday, brought to Washington D.C. on an emergency medivac plane and I should stay in Tulsa and wait. I insisted on talking to the doctor in Germany before making any decisions, so she patched me through. I spoke to Dr. Belin who said that there would not be an emergency flight, although they had considered it so a plasma transfer could be started sooner. Joe was still in a medically induced coma, still on the ventilator, and they had started steroid and anti-viral medications. They were preparing to do a plasma exchange as soon as he got to Bethesda. I didn't know what most of that meant, but what I did know was that I had to get to Germany as soon as possible. After talking to him, I called Donna back and told her that I <u>was</u> getting on the flight and would sort things out with the Marine Corps at a later date.

I called Steven to be sure he was awake, and he assured me that he was getting ready for his flight and would be seeing me soon. That helped calm my nerves. Then it was time to board the plane. The plane to Chicago was a small one and we had to walk outside on the tarmac to the steps leading up to the plane. It was still dark and the air was warm. I was one of the last people in line, possibly THE last one, admiring the moon as I walked, then looking up toward the cockpit. The captain was watching me and we waved to each other. He, on his routine morning flight, and me, off on the adventure of my life.

Meanwhile in Albuquerque, Steven's friend, Kris took him to the airport. He got in the domestic line at the American Airlines check-in and after about 10 minutes, was sent to the International line. After another 10 minutes, he finally got to the front of the line. The first thing the agent asked for was a passport, she seemed upset when he didn't have one and said she could only check his bags as far as Washington D.C., which was what he wanted in the first place. He got his ticket and headed toward the gate. The line at security was long (another 20 minute wait), the flight was already boarding when he got to the gate, and he was the next to last person to get on the plane.

My flight to Chicago was full and I sat by the window, which was nice; watching the sun come up over the horizon, comforted me as the warm, orange rays shined through the clouds. The passenger in the seat next to me began to talk and it occupied my mind. He was a salesman who took the flight to Chicago often, used to live in Springfield and chattered about how the town used to be. He wished me luck as the plane landed and we parted ways.

I left the plane, went to the nearest flight information board to see where my next gate was and was horrified to see that my flight to Washington D. C. had been cancelled! I hurried to the gate and found a line of people, everyone trying to make arrangements for another flight. As I was waiting my turn, the fellow in front of me got to the counter, and then turned to his friend who was in line behind me, motioning him to the counter. Just then a second agent opened another line and motioned me over to her. She started to enter my information in the computer, and then told me that the last two seats had just been filled — with the two guys in the other line. I was stunned! The next flight wasn't until 3:00, which would put me into D. C. after 5:00 pm, and that would be too late to catch the flight to Germany.

Fighting back tears, I explained to her that I had to be there no later than 3:00 in order to make the connection to Germany, and I told her the reason for my trip. She began to type things into her computer and told me that I <u>would</u> be on the next flight to D.C. if she had to put me on the plane herself. I was SO relieved. My original flight was supposed to leave at 10 a.m. and she managed to get me on the 11 a.m. flight. I thanked her again and again, and then called Sgt. Nichols to tell him of the flight change. I had some time to kill so I found a McDonald's that was serving breakfast, got an egg & cheese biscuit, took a couple of Kava Kava to calm my nerves and sat down to wait. Steven's plane was in the air so I left a message on his voice mail. My original flight would have gotten to D. C. about an hour before Steven's flight but now it appeared that he'd be arriving about the same time. Things were working out. Or so I thought.

Steven had a flight change in Dallas, and got my message there; it was going to be more of an adventure than he had planned on.

When 11:00 came and went, I began to get nervous. The departure sign changed to 11:30 and there was no plane at the gate. I took another Kava Kava. Soon the sign changed to 12:00 and I began to pace, no plane at the gate, this was bad. Finally, a plane pulled in and started to unload. The sign changed to 12:30. I took another Kava Kava, paced some more, and called Sgt. Nichols, my Marine liaison, my rock. He also sounded nervous and asked me to call just as soon as my plane landed in D. C. On the flight, I tried to read, tried to be calm, all the while knowing that every minute would count now.

As I sat there on the plane, I tried to remember what Joe had told me in his recent phone calls. He had been feeling bad and his arm had been hurting. I knew that he had gotten the smallpox vaccination a couple of days before leaving the country; he had even asked me if it was possible to get smallpox from the vaccination. He had also had a typhoid vaccination, just two days after the smallpox vaccination.

I wondered if those two vaccinations had anything to do with what was happening to him.

My plane finally touched down at 3:00 at Reagan Airport in Washington D. C., Steven had been there a full hour and a half and I knew he'd be waiting. As the plane taxied toward the gate, I called Sgt. Nichols. He told me that he had talked to Steven and we needed to find our Marine driver as soon as possible. As I briskly walked past the security checkpoint, I could see them both standing at the end of the hall. Thank God. I gathered them up and we hurried to baggage claim. As we were waiting for my bags, a little boy who had been on my plane came over to our (in uniform) Marine driver and asked him if he could shake his hand. "Thank you for what you do", he said. What a breath of fresh air! We all smiled and marveled at the boy's spirit. He was only 5 or 6 years old, and he boosted MY spirits to the moon and stars.

Steven already had his luggage so, as soon as we got my bags, we hurried to the government car which was parked right outside the door, even closer than the taxi cabs. "That's the good thing about government license plates," said our driver, whom we had learned was Sgt. Collins. We loaded up and drove downtown to the passport office, it was going to be close. I had never been to Washington D.C. but, as a history buff, I had always wanted to see the museums there. Unfortunately, we were even too pressed for time for drive-by sight seeing. I had always wanted to visit every state plus D.C. and, at the time, I had just 3 states to go. I didn't know then, but by the end of the day, I would have only one state left on my list — Hawaii. Someday, I hope to go there too.

We got to the passport office just 30 minutes before closing time and the big sign said it would take at least an hour to get a passport. I was afraid the clerk was going to send us away, but he gave us some forms to fill out then started looking at our paperwork. I was horrified when he said I didn't have the proper birth certificate, but a quick phone call later, and he said it would be alright. Then, at 5 minutes till closing, he asked for our photos — nobody had mentioned photos, and we hadn't given it a thought. He sent us to a photographer who just happened to be next door and happened to provide instant passport photos (for a price), and we were back in 10 minutes with them. It was after 4:30 by then, quitting time for the passport office people, but they stayed late to take care of us and at 4:50 the guard let us out a side door, passports in hand.

We located Sgt. Collins, illegally parked (thank goodness for government tags), and talking on his cell phone to his superior. We jumped in the car, hoping to make it to Dulles Airport in time, and in rush hour traffic. For Steven and I, it was a time to relax and get our wits about us but for our driver, it was crunch time. He carefully, but as quickly as possible, got us to the airport and stayed with us until we had checked our bags at the counter. We thanked him for all his help (couldn't have done it without him) and hurried through the security check. We followed the signs to a bus-like vehicle that drove us out to the international terminal, checking in at the gate just 5 minutes before the plane was to begin boarding. Thank you, Lord!

At this point, it suddenly hit us that we had only eaten airplane snacks all day, it was 6:25 p.m., we were about to get on an eight hour flight, and we were starving. Most people would just get on the plane and wait for a meal to be served, but we are both vegetarians and we didn't know if we'd be able to eat what they served. So we asked the lady who checked us in if we could run to the Subway (just a short walk back) for a sandwich. She told us that once we got to the gate we were not allowed to leave (security reasons) but she would give us 5 minutes (we must have looked starved too). If we weren't back

First One Home

in 5 minutes they would pull our bags off the plane. We promised to hurry, walked as quickly as possible, got 2 sandwiches to go, and hurried back. She was paging us as we entered the gate area. We had made it just in time. Two minutes later, the plane began boarding and we followed the crowd to our seats. It was a full plane and they didn't have two seats together but we had aisle seats directly across from each other, close enough to talk. We settled in for the long flight.

When we got in the air, I checked out the movie selection but didn't see anything that looked good so I left the airline information screen on, as we ate our Subway sandwiches. They were sooooo good. When he was finished eating, Steven reached in his backpack and pulled out an itty-bitty tube of toothpaste and a toothbrush.

"Do you like my $3.00 tube of toothpaste?" he asked.

"You know, you could have gotten it for fifty cents if you'd gone to Wal-mart," I answered.

"Well, I had one four times this size that I bought for $1.00 at the dollar store."

"Why didn't you bring it?" I asked.

"I did, but they took it away from me at the security checkpoint in Albuquerque."

"Why would they do that?" I asked, confused.

"Because you can't bring more than 3 ounces on an airplane now. So I had to buy this little guy from the gift shop at the airport," he answered. "I hope I don't have to brush my teeth too many times."

I laughed as he got up, walking to the restroom in the back to brush his teeth. He had become rather obsessive about brushing his teeth, brushing every time he ate, and I knew that he wouldn't have made it without that little tube.

There was a TV screen on the back of each seat on the airplane and, if you didn't select a movie, you could scroll through several information screens. One of the screens was a map with a little airplane to indicate where the plane was and I watched the little plane as it inched its way across the water. I believe that was the slowest little plane I've ever seen! It took forever to clear the U. S. coast, flying northward over a sliver of Canada, then out over the ocean. I thought about the movie "The Perfect Storm" as I recognized the fishing areas where the boat had been trapped.

About an hour into the flight, we were all shocked to hear one of the stewards come on the intercom asking for a doctor or nurse to come to the back of the plane. Rumors started almost immediately, it was an older lady, sick, possibly having a heart attack or maybe a stroke. I looked at the little airplane map, trying to guess where we would land if they had to take her off the plane. My next thought was "This is why I didn't want Lou to come; it could be him having the health problems, out over the ocean with limited medical help available." Instantly, I was glad he was safe at Teri's house.

The doctors on board took care of the lady with the health problem and banished the rest of the passengers from the back of the plane. Dinner came and Steve & I were glad to see there was food we could eat on the tray — we were still hungry — probably nerves, I decided, and took more Kava Kava. They settled my nerves and I kept busy reading the papers I had brought along. Soon, nature called, and I went to find the restroom. Many others had the same idea and there was a line at the forward lavatories. Since the back of the plane was still off limits, everyone from coach had to go forward and use the lavatories in first class. The stewardesses in first class were miffed but what can you do? I waited my turn, and then hurried back to my seat. No need in getting involved in that drama. I watched the movie "The Breakup", and then went back to watching the little plane slowing flying over the big ocean, and my thoughts turned to Joe.

First One Home

Joe had been a good baby, well behaved and a fast learner. He seemed to do everything early, walking and potty trained before his first birthday. He knew all his letters by 18 months, and could read some books by 2 years of age. He had always loved to read and had started making movies in junior high school. I smiled when I remembered some of the films he and his friends had made back then. He also discovered music in junior high, learning to play the drums in the school band. I had been a drummer in junior high school too, and I was pleased when he chose percussion. Joe had played with the marching band in high school and Lou & I went to every competition, spending several weekends a year following the buses and helping cook the meals. He had attended Willard High School, a small town just outside Springfield, Missouri, and the school was known far and wide for their band. They always did well and we spent many long days in the bleachers. Those were the days....

It was during those high school years that Joe learned to love backpacking, hiking, and rock climbing. He also discovered drama, acting in school plays and was even nominated for best comedian in the area during his senior year. It was quite an honor as the nominations were made by his peers. He had always been comical. He combined his humor with many of his videos and had even thought about studying film making in college.

It was early in his senior year of high school that Joe decided to join the Marine Corps. I didn't think he was cut out to be a Marine, he was a little guy — at 5'3" tall, barely meeting the minimum height requirement — and he weighed in at a mere 120 pounds. I was convinced that he would never survive boot camp. I knew that the Marines had the toughest training and tried to talk him into another branch of the service, any other branch. I made him talk to all the recruiters in town. But he had the dream, he had the vision, he wanted to be a Marine. I didn't understand it then, but I would learn. He had the heart, he had the drive to be one of the few, the proud, a Marine. I would catch his vision later, becoming one of the few, the proud myself — a proud Marine Mom.

Joe left for boot camp just 3 days after high school graduation, it was my birthday, May 24, 2004, and I was not thrilled. After 13 long weeks of basic training, Lou, Steven and I went to San Diego for his graduation — and on August 23, 2004, a new Marine was born. He was so handsome in his uniform and we had never been prouder! Joe came home and started college, spending that first school year going to Kansas City once a month for his reserve weekends. The following summer he went to 29 Palms for his MOS training, where he learned to be a radio operator. He had just started his second year of college when Hurricanes Katrina and Rita hit and he volunteered to help. He withdrew from classes, went to New Orleans, got the job done and made it home in time for second semester, but then the call came to go to Iraq. It hadn't been that long ago, but it seemed a lifetime ago.....

We had been in the air for about four hours when the other passengers began to turn off their reading lights and try to sleep. Steven went to sleep but I was wide awake. I decided to go to the back of the plane and try to find something to drink. When I got there, I found a small group of people just standing around. Waiting for the restroom? No, just couldn't sleep. Well, these were my kind of people so I decided to join them. There were about 6 of us and we stood there for the longest time, everyone telling stories about their trips to Germany, and the stewards joining in, laughing and joking with everyone. One of the stewards was gay and the other wasn't and they were joking with each other, and all of us night owls, about which lifestyle was the best. It was such fun. My new friends were all going to Germany for business or vacation, and their stories were great, but my story was the one they were all interested in hearing. They were all very concerned and wished me the best of luck, promising to keep us in their prayers. Even the stewards joined in, they were all so very sweet and caring.

Soon another person joined our group; it was the little lady who had had the health problem soon after take off. As it turned out, she was in her 70's and had had a panic attack. She was taking a trip to see Russia. She was a sweet lady, embarrassed by her attack and the way it had affected the other passengers. We all liked her instantly. What a spunky lady, I thought, going off to Russia at her age. She was a sweetheart.

Eventually, I went back to my seat, and found that Steven was awake and wondering where I'd been for so long. He was afraid I had gotten air sick. We sat and talked quietly so we wouldn't wake the other passengers, until the stewards began serving breakfast. Aaaa, more food, we were hungry again — must be nerves. The little plane on the computer screen finally started flying over land again as we got closer and closer to Frankfort. It was 1:30 a.m. according to my body time, but 9:30 a.m. local time when we landed. I was just beginning to get sleepy but, in Frankfort, the city was just waking up for the day. It must be what people call "jet lag".

Chapter 7

Thursday, October 5

Germany

As we left the airplane, the stewards said goodbye and, once again, wished us well. We stepped into the terminal and I suddenly realized that I was in a foreign place where the signs meant nothing and even the pictures next to the words weren't familiar. Steven and I followed the other passengers, hoping they would lead us in the right direction. But, we soon realized that our fellow passengers were all looking for connecting flights, not baggage claim as we should be. We stopped and reassessed our position, realizing that we had gone past the security checkpoint and would have to go back through.

Luckily, the security people spoke some English and were able to understand that we were lost — and we weren't alone, there were about 10 others from our flight who had done the same thing and were making their way back through security too. We laughed at each other and waited our turn in line.

It didn't take long to see that security checks were different in Germany. Walking through the metal detector and removing shoes was the same but then there was the wand all around the body and the bottom of the feet followed by the pat down. Carry-on items went through the x-ray machine, and as we gathered up our things, Steven turned to me and said "I think I feel violated". Yep, it was a pretty thorough pat-down. We chuckled, deciding not to think about it, trying to concentrate on finding our bags.

We finally saw a sign that looked like a suitcase and followed it into a room where the man behind the counter was looking at a computer screen. As we approached him, he stuck his hand out, never taking his eyes off the screen or uttering a word. I put my passport in his hand, he looked at it, looked at me, stamped a page and handed it back without a word. He put his hand out toward Steven, repeating the process, and then went back to his computer screen. Steven and I looked at each other, not knowing what to do next, then decided the man at the computer must be done with us and continued on, following the suitcase pictures around the corner and into another room. The room looked familiar, with the conveyor belt that luggage travels on, and we soon found our bags. There didn't seem to be anyone in the room who was interested in talking to us, so we assumed we were finished and went to the large doors just opposite the doors we'd used to enter the room, and they slid open in front of us. It had to be the exit.

I took a deep breath as we walked through the exit doors and into the airport terminal, not knowing what would happen next. Sgt. Nichols had told me that someone would meet us at the airport and, sure enough, standing right in front of us were two people in civilian clothes holding signs — one with my name on it and the other with Steven's name — just like in the movies. They introduced themselves as Major Bacon and Sgt. Poor, our Marine Liaisons, and said that they would be driving us to the base where Joe was, about a

45 mile drive. They had a rolling cart for our bags and we piled them on. Steven was wearing his Salvador Dali Museum t-shirt, Major Bacon had visited there and the two of them began talking about it. They were immediately comfortable with each other and were soon chatting like old friends.

As we walked to the parking lot, I noticed the shops in the airport, all different kinds of shops, even a small grocery store. It was very different from American airports. We asked to stop at the restroom and I noticed that the sign said "toilet", not "restroom". As I approached the lady's room door, a man came out. I paused a minute to look at the picture again, thinking that I might have made a mistake, but there was definitely a picture of a woman on the door. Another deep breath and I went in. The first room had sinks and another door lead to the room where the toilets were. Later, as I stopped in the sink room to wash my hands, I noticed another man, standing in the corner writing on a clipboard. It was startling to see men in the ladies room. I asked Major Bacon about it but she just smiled and said "not an unusual thing around here." Must be a German thing.

We proceeded down the hallway toward the parking garage, stopping at a machine on the wall, where Robert (Sgt. Poor) inserted money to pay for parking, then we proceeded out the door. As we entered the parking lot, Steven and I noticed lots of hatchbacks and Mercedes Benz. In fact, the van we got into was a Mercedes. Robert told us that Mercedes were common in Germany, like Fords and Chevies in America. We pulled out of the parking lot and made our way to the autobahn where traffic was at a stand still. We had always heard about the "no speed limit" on the autobahn so this was not expected. Robert, who was driving, told us that traffic would get better when we got outside the city. He was right, as we got further

First One Home

and further away from the city, traffic began to move faster and faster. Soon we were moving right along, past fields of green plants, grapevines, and tall sunflowers. We passed some familiar looking places too, a Wal-Mart Super Center and a McDonalds.

As we drove toward the base, we were given an update on Joe's condition. We learned that he was stable but still in a drug-induced coma. The doctors were planning to fly him to America on either Friday or Tuesday. We drove past an Air Force Base, then into a wooded area and up a winding road, finally stopping at the gate to Landstuhl Army Base. It was in a beautiful forest. Major Bacon called someone on her cell phone and told them that we were at the gate. We got out of the van, went into the guard house, presented our passports, and got our passes. It was a short drive from the gate to the hospital, and Robert pulled right up to the emergency room entrance. He told us that we were meeting the chaplain there and would wait in the van for a minute as it was cold outside. It was clear that we wouldn't be going into the hospital until the chaplain arrived. I was afraid that Joe might have died and the chaplain was going to be the one to tell us. My mind was racing!

Soon the chaplain, Lee, arrived and took all of us inside the hospital, explaining as we walked that Joe would look bad, his body was swollen and he had lots of tubes running in and out of him. I was relieved to hear that he was still alive. Lee said that Joe was still not responding for them. He kept explaining how bad patients in ICU look and it suddenly occurred to me that he was afraid we were going to freak out when we saw him. I assured him that I had been in ICU before, could handle it no matter how bad he looked, and just wanted to get in there to see him.

Joe was in Room 1, the first room on the right as we entered. We could see through the window, but not much. The nurse was doing something with him and Lee told us we'd have to "gown up" while we were waiting. We put on the first of many paper-like tie-in-the-back yellow gowns and plastic gloves. "These are to protect you from any germs he may have brought back with him from Iraq", Lee explained. I could see the bed through the window and strained to see Joe's face as his nurse hovered over him. A doctor approached on my left and introduced himself, telling us that Joe was totally paralyzed and the ventilator was breathing for him. He tried to prepare us for what he would look like with all the machines around him. He said that Joe had tried to open his eyes once or twice, but mostly had not been responding to them. I just wanted to get into the room.

I had entered my "mother bear" mode, like a momma bear protects and watches over her cubs, I was ready for anything. I was ready to fight for my little cub, just bring it on, I was ready. I was tough; nothing was going to get in my way now. I had become the momma bear.

I had been in the "mother bear" mode a few times before; in fact, I remembered a time twenty years earlier, when I was pregnant with Joe, and became the momma bear. Steven had gone out with his skateboard, fell, and sliced his chin open (he still has the scar). He came into the house holding his chin, blood dripping out between his fingers, saying "I'm OK, I'm OK". The momma bear marched him right into the bathroom, rinsed off his chin, applied pressure with a clean towel and shouted for Lou to get the car keys. Lou was an odd shade of gray and stood leaning against the wall but somehow got it together enough to get to the car. He knew better than to mess with the momma bear.

I suppose we were quite a sight as we went rushing into the emergency clinic: dad pale and falling into the nearest chair; 10 year old Steven insisting he didn't need stitches; and momma bear,

8 months pregnant, holding that white towel as it slowly turned to red. Yes, I'm sure we were quite a sight! The nurse showed us to a room right away (not Lou, he stayed where he was) and brought me a chair but I didn't sit down. The doctor came in and begged me to sit, "I'm afraid you might faint when I start stitching this up," he said. Obviously, he had not met the momma bear before, the weak knees wouldn't come until well after the stitching was over — and the bear cub was safe at home, sleeping peacefully in his own bed……..

The nurse blocked our way as we tried to enter the ICU room. "I've turned down the medication that is keeping him in the coma" she said, "he should start becoming more alert in a few minutes. We want you to talk to him so we can see if he'll react." Steven and I both nodded, and she stepped out of the way. We would learn that the medication she was talking about was nicknamed "milk of amnesia" as it was white in color and one of the side effects is that the patients don't remember the worst parts of their illnesses.

I went to the right side of the bed and Steven went to the left side, and as soon as I saw Joe I knew why the doctors had been so concerned. Most of his body was covered with blankets but I could see that his face and hands were swollen dramatically. He had tubes running in and out of his body: the vent tube in his mouth, a feeding tube in his nose, I.V. lines under both collar bones and in both arms, a urine bag hanging on the side of the bed, and the round EKG pads pressed onto his chest. I could see that the I.V.s were pumping several different medications into his body along with a saline solution. His head was held still by sponge-like squares on either side and the bed was moving as air was pumped in then out of it, moving his body from side to side to keep bedsores from forming. The machines made beeping and whirling sounds. Yes, he was quite a sight to see, and momma bear took his hand gently. After a few minutes, the nurse nodded and said, "Try talking to him now."

I leaned in ever so slightly and said "Hi, Joe, it's mom. I'm here." In an instant, he opened both eyes, shut them, and then opened them again! I don't remember what I said next, but as soon as he heard my voice, he opened his eyes again. I could hear the nurse catch her breath.

Steven leaned in next and said "Hi Joe, it's Steve and I'm here too." Once again, his eyes flew open, and then closed. The nurse whispered "YES!", and the doctor said "Alright, that's good." Both of them were smiling as they left the room and we could hear them talking, in excited tones, in the hallway. We stayed for about half an hour, talking to Joe, telling him where he was, what had happened, and what was going to happen. We didn't know how much he was hearing, or understanding, but we kept talking. Then his nurse came in, said she needed to adjust his medication and do some other things with him but we could come back later. It was a gentle hint, time for us to go.

As we left the room, we saw that Major Bacon was gone but Robert was still waiting, so we took off our yellow gowns and gloves and left ICU with him. I was relieved to have seen Joe and to know that he was alive. We got back into the van and Robert took us to the Fisher House, where they apologized because there was only one room available. The room had twin beds in it and we were glad to get it. I didn't want to be alone anyway; it would be good to have Steven nearby.

We learned that the Fisher House is run with donations and provided to the families free of charge. Our room was on the 2nd floor and had its own bathroom. There was a kitchen area on the 1st floor, fully stocked with pans and dishes and a store room full of

First One Home

food. There was a refrigerator and freezer that were full of food too. We could have anything we wanted to eat, as long as we cleaned up after ourselves. There was a dining room, a living room with a big screen TV and two computers that we could use. It was a very nice place. There were international telephone calling cards in our room, so I made a quick call to Teri using one of them. We put our bags in our room then went with Robert to the chow hall. I don't remember what time of day it was but they were starting to put the food away as lunch time was over. I made a quick trip to the salad bar and Steven found some vegetables. Robert left us for a few minutes but came back about the time we were finished eating. He told us that we were his only job while we were there.

We went back to ICU and met Joe's doctor, Dr. McMahon, who told us that they were planning to transport Joe on the medivac plane the next morning. I was concerned that he might not be strong enough to make such a long trip but the doctor assured us that, not only was he stable enough but he needed to get to Bethesda as soon as possible as they didn't have the medicine they needed to treat him with in Germany.

I noticed that there was a small blanket and t-shirt on the shelf in Joe's room, and unfolded them to get a better look. "Nice blanket," I said to Steven "looks homemade, like a miniature quilt." I had noticed a small blanket in our room at the Fisher House too. We didn't know the story behind the blankets, but would learn later that they are made by volunteers and each patient is given one. They use them to cover their legs to keep them warm on the flight home, a little something from home — a security blanket in every sense of the word.

Robert took us back to the Fisher House so we could unpack our bags, shower, and send some e-mails. It was cold and drizzling rain.

While we were there, we met the Sharps; their son had been wounded in Iraq by an IED. They were also staying at the Fisher house, and were standing just outside the front door, smoking cigarettes, both wearing Marine sweatshirts. They told us that they had been in Germany for a week and their son, who was 19 years old, would also be flying out on Friday.

When we got back to the hospital, we met the flight surgeon and a couple of others who would be on the hospital plane with Joe the next day. They told us that the plane was specially outfitted to transport the wounded, keeping them as comfortable as possible. The medivac planes are sterile like a hospital and equipped to do surgery while in flight, if necessary. To make it easier on the patients, they don't fly as high as commercial planes and they also fly slower, so it takes about 2 hours longer for them to get to Washington D.C. They told us that we could fly on the medivac plane if there was room, but the flight was full, so we would have to fly commercial. Joe was heavily sedated but we talked to him anyway, just in case he could hear us. I used one of the phone cards to call Teri's house from the phone next to Joe's bed — and put the phone next to his ear so Lou could talk to him. I didn't know if Joe could hear him, but it made Lou feel better.

The nurses told us that the Commandant and Sgt. Major of the Marine Corps were in the hospital and had been visiting the patients in ICU. We learned that they had been there when Steven & I had first arrived and had looked in the door. They didn't want to disturb us, as we were trying to get Joe to respond to us, so they didn't come in. The Sgt. Major had seen Joe the previous day, and they were both concerned about his condition. It was comforting to know that the top two men in the Marine Corps had traveled to Germany and were looking in on the wounded.

All too soon, it was time for the nurses to work with Joe, and Robert took us back to the Fisher House. Steven and I were extremely tired but also very hungry and decided to check out the kitchen. A box of macaroni and cheese looked good, so we found a pot and started cooking; Steven used the computer to send more e-mails while I finished our "gourmet" dinner. We divided the macaroni onto two plates, went to the dining area to eat, and enjoyed the best mac & cheese ever. While we were eating, a man came in the front door and stopped to talk to us. His name was Johnson and his son was also a Marine. He had been in Germany for three days but his son was not yet stable enough to fly. He hoped that they would be able to leave on the Tuesday flight and promised to look us up when he got to Bethesda.

I'm not sure when we got to bed that night, but I know it was well after midnight, Germany time, which would have been early evening "my body time". I tried to figure it, since getting up to go to work on Tuesday — about 60 hours ago — I had slept about 5 hours — no wonder I was so tired! Robert was coming to pick us up at 7:00 a.m. That meant we would have about 5 hours of sleep, so we set the alarm and, even though we were in a strange place and in strange beds, we were both asleep as soon as our heads hit the pillows. It was a good sleep.

Chapter 8

Friday, October 6

The Flight to Bethesda

The alarm went off at 6 a.m. and Steven and I got dressed, packed our bags, and had a quick bowl of cereal in the kitchen. We were tired, but wanted to see Joe again before we left for Frankfurt and our flight home. Robert picked us up at 7:00 sharp and took us to the hospital. It was still cold and drizzling as we showed our passes to the security guard at the door and started down the hall toward ICU. We had decided that Robert was an amazing guy. He'd stayed with us until after midnight, driven to his home off base, then came back to get us at 7 a.m. It was good to have someone like him looking after us.

The airplane crew was in ICU when we got there, getting information on each patient and preparing them for the flight. There was a different crew for each patient and the ICU was bustling with activity. Joe's team gave us a few minutes with him as they worked to get the portable equipment ready. We knew he'd be unhooked from the machines in his room and hooked up the portable equipment soon. We talked to him, not knowing if he could hear us, for he was deep in the induced coma. Soon it was time for us to go and we each kissed his forehead and told him we'd see him soon. It was hard to leave him, knowing we wouldn't see him for half a day and not until we had all traveled halfway around the world. We knew that he would be placed on a gurney, loaded into a bus-type ambulance, driven to the Air Force base we'd passed the day before, and loaded onto the hospital plane. We also knew that the plane would land at Andrews Air Force Base and he'd be transported to Bethesda Naval Hospital from there. We expected him to get there before us. It was time to go.

We made our way to the emergency room entrance and found Robert and the Sharps waiting in the van. It was 7:30 as we left for the Frankfurt Airport. The ride to the airport was a quiet one; everyone was still half asleep, and worried about our boys. The day before, I had asked Robert about buying some souvenirs, but the hospital gift shop had already closed. He had located a coffee cup with the hospital logo on it that morning, and gave it to me during our drive; it was the only thing we brought back from Germany. We finally got to the airport, and made our way inside. The Marine liaisons had booked all of us on the same plane, but when we went to get our boarding passes, we learned that our flight (leaving at 10 a.m.) had been cancelled. Just my luck! Another cancelled flight. Robert was able to get the Sharps on a noon flight to Munich, where they could make a connection to Washington D.C., and they slipped away to smoke.

Steven and I were told that we'd have to go on different flights, or wait until 5:00 pm, with one of us flying standby. We weren't happy with that, so Robert talked to another agent who found two seats on the 11:00 non-stop flight, if we could get to the gate in time. We got our boarding passes and Robert showed us to the customs area.

Steven was given a Ziploc bag for his tiny toothpaste and I got one for my lipstick. "I think my baggie looks like it has more in it than yours," I joked.

There was one long line of people which split into 10 or 12 other lines just past the first check point, then each of those lines had an x-ray machine for carry-on baggage. Robert pointed out that most people were going into the nearby lines and the lines to the far left were much shorter. He wanted to check on the Sharps so we told him goodbye and thanked him for everything he'd done for us — just in case we were past the ropes when he came back. As soon as we got in front of the ropes, we hurried to the line that was the farthest to the left and got through very quickly. After showing our passports and being cleared to go into the terminal, we turned to see if Robert had returned but he wasn't there. The plane was boarding and we had to hurry. We never saw our friend Robert again.

Steven and I got to the gate just as the last passengers were starting down the walkway. We were the last ones to board the plane. The plane was a 767, just like the one we'd flown in on, and the flight attendants looked very familiar — it was the same plane and the same crew, on their return trip to Washington. I think they were as surprised to see us as we were to see them, and one of them stopped me to ask how my son was doing. It was bizarre but comforting.

Since we had gotten the last two seats on the plane, Steven and I weren't sitting together but we were in the same row. We were surrounded by a group of ladies who had been touring Europe together and were on their way home. They were a happy group, and had obviously had a great time on their trip. It soon became apparent to them that we were traveling together and the lady sitting next to me offered to change places with Steven so she could be sitting closer to her friends and Steve and I could sit together too. It was a win-win situation for everyone.

Steven and I had time to talk about what we'd seen in Germany during the flight, and we were fortunate to get lunch and a snack, both of which had food that we could eat. Later, as Steven slept, I got out the bills I'd brought with me and wrote out checks. I also looked at some of the reading material I'd brought along. One of the articles I read was about a young Marine from Columbia, MO who had been injured a week earlier, 2 weeks now, in Iraq. I made a mental note to look for him when we got to Bethesda and put the article back in my bag. I watched Pirates of the Caribbean, and then switched to Cars. I'd heard that it was a good kid's movie and it put me to sleep right away. When I woke up, the movie had started to play again, so I watched the ending. I suddenly realized that I hadn't taken any Kava Kava for my nerves since I'd walked into Joe's hospital room at Landstuhl. I guess the nerves calm down and calmness sets in when the momma bear takes over.

The plane landed at 2 p.m. at Dulles Airport and I felt refreshed after my nap. As we were taxiing toward the terminal, the lady sitting beside me apologized for the group she was traveling with. She felt bad that they'd been having such a good time while I was going through such a hard time with my son. She also wanted me to know how much they appreciated what he and the other troops were doing for our country. I assured her that they had not offended me and that it was actually good for me to see people having a good time. It had raised my spirits to see such happy people. She was so nice. All the ladies who were sitting near us said they would keep us (and Joe) in their prayers. As we exited the plane, the crew also wished us luck and promised to pray for Joe.

As we waited for our bags, we remembered the scene in the Die Hard movie that was filmed in the same baggage claim area. It was fun to be in a place that we'd seen in the movies. We got through customs and headed toward the entrance, keeping our eyes open for someone in a Marine uniform who might be there to pick us up. We weren't sure what would happen, since we'd been put on a different flight and even though Robert had said he'd let someone know, we weren't sure if it would work out. We also knew that the Sharps had left an hour behind us and thought they might pick us all up at the same time. When we didn't find anyone, I called Sgt. Nichols, and learned that there was a driver from Bethesda who was on the way but was delayed by traffic and the weather (it was cold and misting). I told him which door we were near, and we sat down to watch for a likely vehicle.

It was nearly 4 p.m. when I a van pulled into the loading zone and a Marine in fatigues got out. I walked over to him and he confirmed that he was, indeed there for us, so we brought our bags to the van. Our driver was named Martin and I think he was a Lance Corporal, like Joe. He said he also had the Sharp's names but their flight had been delayed so someone else would pick them up. We noticed the scars on his left arm right away and Steven asked him what had happened. He told us that he had been wounded by an IED in his left arm and leg while serving in Iraq. He had had 28 surgeries on his arm over the past 7 months, and had just finished physical therapy on his leg. We were in the midst of rush hour traffic but Martin, who was from the D. C. area, knew of a few shortcuts. He made several turns and soon we were out of the stop-and-go traffic. Steven had struck up a friendship with him and had started calling him the Transporter, as he transported people around the city and also because he had been a Marine Corps driver before his injury. As we drove through

First One Home

the front gate at Bethesda Naval Medical Center, I recognized the tower building immediately, as I had seen it many times in pictures and movies. I had no way of knowing that I wouldn't go out that gate for nearly two months.

Martin took us directly to the Navy Lodge, a motel run by the Navy on base. It was located about ¾ of a mile from the hospital and was directly behind the two Fisher Houses, both of which were full. Martin waited for us to check in and put our bags in our room, and then he drove us to the hospital. He showed us to the Marine Liaison office, located on the first floor, near the entrance of Building 10, where we met SSgt. Perez, the liaison assigned to us. We learned that Joe had arrived, been admitted to ICU, and was currently having an MRI. He also told us that the hospital dining room was closed, but since it was Friday night, there was a special dinner, free of charge, and just for the families of the wounded, in the executive dining room. The dinner had already started and they were serving Philippine food. Neither of us had ever had Philippine food but we were hungry and decided to try it.

We went down the elevator to the basement, made a wrong turn, and were halfway to the morgue before we realized where we were going. Oh, no, better not go there. We spun around and found our way to the executive dining room. The room was very nice, with three long tables and comfortable chairs, enough to sit 60 or 70 people, and a big screen TV at the far end. I imagined the room being used by officers for working lunches.

When we arrived, we were greeted by a very lovely lady, the top person in the cafeteria as it turned out. She made us feel very welcome, and made sure we got all the food we could eat. We would see her several more times over the next few weeks, she always recognized us and knew how many times we had come to the Friday night dinners.

The food was quite good. We had white rice, mixed vegetables, fried vegetable rolls and fried plantains for dessert.

After dinner, we went back to the liaison office where SSgt. Perez showed us around the office, pointing out the refrigerator where we could help ourselves to bottled water or Gatorade. There was also a storage area with toiletries (tiny toothpaste, shampoo, etc.) and clothing (T-shirts, sweatshirts, etc.) which we could take, if we needed anything. I pointed out the toothpaste to Steven but he said he thought he'd get a bigger tube at the BX. Even if it's a $3.00 tube for free? He just laughed.

Next, SSgt. Perez took us to ICU, which was on the third floor, also in Building 10, and we found Joe in Room 5, near the nurse's station. There was a computer just outside his door where the nurses could enter all his information. We met Dr. King, the doctor on duty, and he told us that Joe had tolerated the flight well but was still sedated. We had to put on the same yellow gown, gloves, and now, a mask before we went into the room. I wasn't thrilled about wearing the mask; it made me claustrophobic, so I pulled it off as often as possible. If the doctors or nurses saw me, they'd ask me to put it back on.

I noticed the same blanket and t-shirt that we'd seen in Joe's room in Germany; and it was comforting to know that they had been with him the whole day. Joe didn't appear to be any worse even though he'd been flown half way around the world, and we stayed for several hours, mostly watching him sleep.

When Steven & I finally decided to go back to our room at the Navy Lodge, we thought about asking for a ride at the Liaison office, but decided to walk instead. It was a nice walk, about 15 minutes long, in the cool evening air, and it gave us time to talk about the events of the day. The walk seemed to be good for us — and calming.

First One Home

We were in Room 119, which was a nice size room with two queen sized beds, and a kitchenette with a small refrigerator, stove and sink. It was in a quiet location near the end of the hall on the first floor. We made note of the laundry, on the same floor, we knew we would need it soon. We unpacked our bags and I took a quick shower. When I came out Steven was sound asleep. It didn't take long for me to fall asleep too.

Chapter 9

Saturday, October 7

First Day of Treatment

It was the first good night's sleep we'd had in nearly a week. The thought of having Joe back in the States and able to receive treatment; plus the days of little or no sleep had finally caught up with us. As it turned out, taking my shower the night before was the best idea, because Steven ended up with a lukewarm shower in the morning. I guess they neglected to tell us about the hot water problem. It was a rude awakening for him, but we were determined that it wouldn't ruin our day. We walked to the hospital, enjoying the walk again, noting the pretty trees, flowers, and even a stream along the way. Things we wouldn't have seen from a car. We enjoyed the walk and the fresh air.

Since it was a weekend, the galley (cafeteria to us non-military types) and food court in the hospital were both closed. The only eating place open was a Subway in the basement and we were pleased to discover that they had breakfast sandwiches. The sandwiches were quite good, scrambled eggs, cheese, and your choice of veggies. We didn't know it at the time, but we would become frequent customers of this Subway.

We hurried to Joe's ICU room, where he was being examined by Dr. Watson, a neurologist. We also met Dr. Montgomery, a Navy immunologist, one of only four. We didn't know it at the time, but he would turn out to be the one we would lean on the most. He was very likeable and had a way of "dumbing down" the medical terms so we could understand them ….. without making us feel like total idiots. He was always ready with an answer, a joke, and a smile and I suspected that he would make a great teacher.

Dr. Montgomery explained that, although they had considered other things along the way (including Guillain-Barre and Multiple Sclerosis), Joe's final diagnosis was ADEM. ADEM stands for Acute Disseminated Encephalomyelitis and it can have several different triggers. Joe's trigger appeared to have been the smallpox vaccination he received just before going to Iraq. He explained that, since the military resumed giving smallpox vaccinations in 2002, less than 1% had experienced adverse reactions. Approximately half of these reactions were in first time vaccinees and occurred within one week of the vaccination. Only 15% of those with adverse reactions experienced serious, life threatening reactions — and only three of those reactions had been ADEM.

Apparently, the smallpox vaccine looks a lot like the nerve endings in the central nervous system and, in ADEM, the person's antibodies not only attack the smallpox but also their own nerves. Joe's antibodies had literally been eating away the myelin sheath (covering) on his nerves. When the myelin gets destroyed enough, the nerves can no longer transmit signals and that is when the numbness begins. The first treatment, high doses of steroids, had failed, which left two other choices, and the two doctors disagreed as to which one was best.

The neurologists, including Dr. Watson, believed that plasma pharesis was the treatment of choice. With this treatment, the patient's blood is removed and run through a machine where the plasma is removed, then replaced with new plasma. In my mind, I pictured a machine similar to a kidney patient's dialysis machine.

Dr. Montgomery explained that the other option was an IV infusion of gammagobulin (other people's antibodies). The doctors believe that the new antibodies either "teach" the old ones how to behave or actually kill them off. They aren't sure which. Either way, the end result is that the destruction of the myelin sheath is stopped and the nerves begin to heal themselves. The other three cases of ADEM had all been treated with plasma pharesis, with varying degrees of success, as each patient lived longer than the last one. The IV gammagobulin (IVIG) had been used with ADEM patients in Europe, but Joe would be the first in the military to be treated with it in America, if we chose that option. After hearing the pros and cons of each treatment, Steven and I talked it over and decided on the IVIG.

Dr. Montgomery's plan was for Joe to get 3 bottles of gammagobulin over 28 hours, a dose that was normally given over 4 days. He would also slowly decrease the steroids over several weeks until they could safely discontinue them. Joe was no longer in a coma, but still mostly sedated. But doctors explained that there were no promises, Joe might wake up or he might not. If he did wake up, the nerve endings in his brain might be too damaged and he could be a vegetable; or his brain could be fine and his body paralyzed. It was scary to hear.

We learned that IVIG was a very expensive treatment, $4,000.00 for each bottle — a total of $12,000.00 for each treatment. IVIG had only been in use for 20 years and the sooner treatment was started, the better the results. They would start the first bottle as soon as they could get it from the pharmacy. Joe would be watched very closely for adverse reactions, especially since the treatment would be given over such a short time period. The worst case scenario would be a shut down of the kidneys or liver. Dr. Montgomery asked us to be there for at least the first few hours, to help the nursing staff watch for reactions — hives, convulsions, fever, and headaches.

Steven and I were overwhelmed by the information the doctors had given us and we left the ICU unit to take time to absorb it all. We stopped at the restrooms on our way back, and Steven called me into the men's room. "What?" I said, "I can't go in there." "You have to see this," he said. I hesitantly peeked in the door, and there on the floor were two pennies. Not one but two lucky pennies. He picked them up, handed them to me, and I put them in the special container I was using to collect my lucky coins. It was another sign.

We went back to Subway, around 1:30, for a late lunch and discovered that they had personal pan pizza. Neither of us had ever had pizza from Subway so we decided to try it — and it was very good. The veggie pizza was a cheese pizza topped with your choice of veggies. This had become a good place for a couple of vegetarians. We had a little time to kill and decided to check out the BX, which was within walking distance. SSgt. Perez had given us a letter which enabled us to shop without a military I.D., we chose a couple of fleece jackets to wear on cool evenings then hurried back to the hospital for the start of the gammagobulin. As the healing fluid began to flow into his veins, we watched Joe for the adverse reactions described to us, but he did well, sleeping peacefully.

After several hours of IVIG treatment, we finally felt comfortable enough to leave Joe to get a bite to eat. While we were out, we saw Mr. Sharp who told us that his son had been in surgery for a good part of the day. He had extensive injuries from the IED which had pretty much destroyed most of one side of his body, including massive wounds to his abdomen.

Lou had called at least a dozen times during the day, each time unable to remember having called before. I explained to him, over and over, where I was and why I was there. He wanted to know when I was coming home, and I tried to explain to him how sick Joe was, and why I couldn't leave him. It was frustrating for me. While we were eating, I called one last time and talked to Teri, making sure she knew what was happening so she could explain it to Lou — once again. I needed her to take care of him, so I could take care of Joe.

Back home, in Springfield, it was the day of the annual high school band competition at Missouri State University. Joe's high school band always competed and usually placed well; and we had spent the day at the football stadium, watching the bands every year for the past 6 years — until this year. I had seen the Willard band perform just one week earlier — a lifetime ago — and I called my friend, Shelia, whose 2 kids were still in the band, to see how they were doing. I learned that the band had taken first place in preliminaries and were waiting to perform in finals. I thought, "When Joe wakes up, he'll be so happy." The band always worked hard for the MSU competition and I would learn later that the Willard band had taken first place in the finals too.

We hurried back to ICU for the gammagobulin bottle change at 11 p.m. then stayed with Joe until well after midnight, watching for adverse reactions, but all went well. Finally, with a sigh of relief, we left for the Navy Lodge.

When we had arrived in Joe's room that morning, we noticed his military backpack sitting in the corner with a Red Cross tag on it. We hadn't noticed it in Germany but knew that it must have come with him on the medivac plane, so we took it back to the Lodge with us. It felt good to have this piece of him with us.

It was nearly 1 a.m. and chilly, and we were glad to have the jackets we'd bought at the BX. We were bone tired again. We talked quietly as we walked along the dimly lit sidewalk. Suddenly, Steven stopped, grabbed my arm and motioned for me to be quiet. Then he pointed ahead of us and I turned to look. Just ahead, a few feet off the sidewalk and directly under a light, there was a deer feasting on the grass under a tree. We stood there for several minutes watching her, she looked up at us a couple of times, and then went back to her meal. She was aware of our presence but was not afraid. After a few minutes, she straightened up, looked at us again, and then ambled off across the road. She was so calm, could this be another sign? We were amazed at what we'd just seen.

We continued up the hill, quietly talking again, past the Fisher Houses, around the corner and into the Navy Lodge parking lot. Steven stopped again, and I followed his gaze to the front yard of an apartment next to the lodge building. There, in the front yard were two more deer, one with antlers, grazing directly under a bird feeder. They looked at us as we started walking again, apparently not afraid even though we were only about 30 feet away from them. We stood at the Lodge entrance and watched them for a few minutes before going inside. It was surely a sign.

In our room, we opened Joe's pack, not knowing what we'd find. He would tell us later that he'd packed for a 1 or 2 day stay at the hospital in Fallujah (who knew?) and had brought books to read, some clothes, his IPOD (but not the charger), and his eyeglasses. We decided to take the glasses back to the hospital in the morning, thinking that he'd be glad to be able to see when he woke up. His dog tags were also there, and I put them around my neck. I would continue to wear them everyday while we were at Bethesda, a ritual that most of the wives/girlfriends/mothers at the hospital followed. They comforted me.

It had been a very eventful day and we were soon sound asleep.

Chapter 10

Sunday, October 8

Near Death

Since we didn't get to sleep until nearly 2 a.m., Steven and I slept late. As I listened to the shower running, I marveled at all that had happened in our lives since that fateful phone call just one week earlier. Who would have ever guessed that something like this would happen to people like us? Who would have guessed how quickly our lives would be turned upside down? Who could predict what would come next? As we walked to the hospital, we talked about the deer who were long gone and marveled at how amazing it was to have seen them.

We were greeted with chaos at the hospital. Joe was beginning to wake up but he was having trouble breathing and they were afraid he might have a blood clot in his lung. The nurses had stopped the IVIG drip and they were preparing him for a CAT scan. We stayed with him until they rolled his bed out the back door of the ICU unit. Steven & I couldn't go with him, so we went to Subway for lunch, taking our time so we wouldn't have to wait in his empty room.

We were shocked when we returned to Joe's room and saw that it was full of doctors and nurses. As we stood at the door, gowning up and trying to figure out what was happening, we noticed that the stool bag hanging on the side of the bed appeared to have blood in it. Dr. T was the resident ICU doctor on duty and he explained that Joe was bleeding internally and they were preparing to do a blood transfusion. I had to sign for it, just as I had signed for the CAT scan earlier that morning. Dr. T suspected the bleeding was in his stomach since the blood was in the stool. I asked him if the IVIG could have caused it, but he said he didn't think so, he suspected a bleeding ulcer. He had called for a G.I. Team to come and run a scope into the stomach but they hadn't arrived yet.

We had been in the room for some time when I heard the nurse on the phone calling the pharmacy; apparently, the blood was ready but there was nobody there to bring it over. The nurse left the unit to go get it herself. When she returned, she had 4 units of blood and 2 units of plasma. She quickly hooked up the first bag of blood and got it running into Joe's IV. She stood there squeezing that bag of blood until it was all gone, making it run into Joe's veins as fast as possible. During that time she would periodically take one hand off the bag, put it at her side and shake it, as if trying to get the blood flowing back into her hand. I could tell that it was hard work for her. She started the second bag, and then went to the nurse's station.

Since Joe's room was very close to the nurse's station, and I was sitting close to the door, I could hear what they were saying very well. I heard Dr. T tell the nurse to call the G.I. Team again and to tell them that it was an emergency. Every time we asked, we were told that the G.I. Team was on the way and would be there shortly. We were told that they were an hour away, 30 minutes away, not very far, almost here, will be here at 5:00, etc., etc. I had started writing a journal and tried to keep busy with that as we waited, but I was getting more and more agitated.

I had known that it was a holiday weekend, but hadn't realized how that seemingly benign fact would affect Joe and his treatment. I hadn't known how close to death he would come just because of the holiday. Now I was beginning to realize that a holiday weekend means a skeleton staff, and that can be dangerous in a hospital setting. There was a problem getting the blood from the pharmacy because of it, and now, it seemed that there was nobody from the G. I. Department in the hospital at all. They were all off for the holiday — Columbus Day.

I've heard that nights, evenings and especially holidays are dangerous times to be in the hospital. I've even heard of studies that have shown patients are more likely to die at these times, but I'd never been confronted with it. The fact is that hospitals are run with a skeleton staff during those times, and those with more seniority (and experience) know to ask early for time off, so the staff on duty for holiday weekends tends to be the most inexperienced. As the day wore on, I became increasingly agitated and concerned that Joe could actually DIE because it was a holiday! How ironic that this young Marine would survive paralysis and coma in the middle of a desert battlefield only to make it to America and bleed to death because of a holiday. Before long, I was furious! The full wrath of the mother bear was about to be unleashed.

Soon the night crew began to come on duty, it was 6:30. The night crew began to tell me things that the day crew hadn't (afraid maybe? told not to say?). I found out, in short order, that the G.I. team wasn't coming at all that night, and that the bleeding was probably a bleeding ulcer caused by a combination of high steroids and too much blood thinner. I asked to speak to Dr. T before he went off duty and found that he was already half way to the door — he wasn't even going to talk to me before he left. I was livid and let him know it right off. He acted surprised that I felt like he hadn't kept me informed.

"That's bullshit and you know it! It's been over 6 hours since this drama began and over 4 hours since you've uttered a word to me. During that time I've heard you say, 'tell them it's an emergency', 'tell him it's urgent', and 'it's about time to step things up'. My son could have died today." I spat out the words as if they were daggers.

"Yes, very easily," he replied

"I waited for hours for you to get someone here to do something and you don't even talk to me before you go off duty?"

"I can't force them to come because they outrank me," he said as he shrugged his shoulders.

That was the wrong thing to say. I could feel the heat in my cheeks, and knew that my face was beet red.

"I don't give a goddamn who outranks you! My child isn't going to die because you are too chicken-shit to do your job. Be a man! And to make matters worse, all this time you were letting my son bleed to death, the healing medicine being pumped into his veins was also bleeding out. Can you guarantee that no permanent damage has been done?"

"No, I can't guarantee that."

"I want to talk to Dr. Montgomery and I'm not signing for any more procedures without talking to him first because I've lost all confidence in the rest of you so-called doctors. Dr. Montgomery is the only one who keeps me informed and doesn't try to feed me a bunch of bullshit!" I had never been so angry!

Dr. T apologized for not keeping me informed and said, "I want him to live as much as you do."

That was like throwing salt on an open wound!

"That's the biggest pile of horse shit you've come up with yet! Who the hell do you think you're talking to? I'm the MOTHER; there isn't anyone on this entire planet who wants that boy to live as much as I do. This time next year, you won't even remember his name. Don't you even TRY to go there with me! Who the hell do you think you are?" I was furious and mama bear was ready to fight!

Once again Dr. T apologized and finally agreed to call Dr. Montgomery. Anything to get away from the furious little woman standing in front of him. As he left to use the phone, Steven came out of Joe's room. He said that Joe was waking up and seemed to be upset by the commotion in the hall.

"Yes, this guy almost killed him, he should be upset," was my response. I know he heard me but Dr. T just kept on walking. I hated for Joe to be waking up and have to see this, but I knew that it had to be done.

While Dr. T was at the nurse's desk calling Dr. Montgomery, Joe's night nurse, Scotty, took me aside to try to calm me down. I liked Scotty, he was a tell-it-like-it-is guy and I didn't think he'd lie to me. He was also a civilian worker, so he didn't have to worry about military politics, like Dr. T (still a resident) obviously did. Soon Dr. T returned, said he'd talked to Dr. Montgomery who had told him that he thought there was still enough IVIG in Joe's blood to do the job and he didn't want to give any extra. He had also talked to the G.I. Team and they had promised to be there at 7 am the next morning. He said that they all felt the danger was over and Joe would do fine overnight.

Dr. Montgomery was on the phone so I went and talked to him. He offered to come in if I wanted him too, but he said he thought Joe was stable at that point. We agreed that he would leave word for the nurses to contact him during the night if anything changed and I knew that Scotty would be watching over him, so we left it at that. Scotty had already promised to keep a good watch during the night and call me if there were any changes at all. Joe seemed to be resting well, Steven thought I needed to calm down, and he talked me into taking a walk outside.

As we left the building, I checked my cell phone and found that Lou had called 5 times! I really didn't need that. I called him back and told him that he had to quit calling me. Once again, I explained to him that Joe was in bad shape and I couldn't take phone calls in ICU. His next question was "when do you think he'll be ready to come home?" I knew he didn't understand, but I couldn't take the pressure anymore. I told him that he couldn't call me anymore, but promised that I would call him every time I left ICU. I think it hurt his feelings, but he finally seemed to get it.

I asked to talk to Teri and told her what had just happened. I broke down and cried when I told her how close Joe had come to dying. She agreed to help me with Lou by trying to get him to stop calling. I knew he was a handful for her but I just couldn't worry about him right then. It was comforting to have Steven with me, and we walked to the Lodge together. Both of us were emotionally spent. We started the laundry and Steven stayed to finish it while I walked back to the hospital alone.

When I got back to the hospital, Joe was sleeping, poor kid. Scotty explained how the high steroids could cause ulcers to form in the stomach and the blood thinners, given for the possible blood clot, could cause the ulcers to bleed uncontrollably. He assured me that Joe was doing well. Soon Steven arrived and we watched Joe sleep until the blood and plasma transfusions were finished, unaware of yet another problem developing.

Joe's feeding tube had become blocked and the nurses had been trying to clear it all day. Scotty said he didn't want to remove the tube unless he absolutely had to and asked if it would be OK to put some Pepsi down it. Apparently, Pepsi is known to unclog feeding tubes. Who knew? I told him that Joe would probably LOVE to have some Pepsi. So he put about half a can of Pepsi through the feeding tube, Joe seemed to like it and it cleared out the tube. What an easy fix. The bleeding seemed to have stopped and they were getting ready to give Joe 2 more units of plasma as Steven & I left for the Lodge. I left my cell phone number with Scotty and he promised to call if anything changed. At some point during the night the IVIG finished.

Chapter 11

Monday, October 9

Columbus Day

Scotty got off work at 7 am, so I sat my alarm for 6:45, and called him. He said that Joe was still bleeding a little bit but seemed to have had a good night other than that. I was relieved to hear it. At 7 am, the G. I. Doctor, Dr. Gentry, called to get my approval to do the endoscopy. I asked him what the point was, now that he'd survived almost bleeding to death and seemed to be improving. He explained that they needed to see what was going on and cauterize any spots that were still bleeding. He also said that there had probably been too much blood in the stomach for them to have done a cauterization the day before. I felt like that was more bullshit, but let it go, and gave my authorization for the scope. He called me back an hour later to say that they were finished and Joe had done well. They found six spots that had been bleeding and had cauterized one of them.

On our way to the hospital, we ran into Mr. Sharp, who told us that his son was in surgery again. This time they were amputating one of his legs which had become infected. He was understandably sad about it, but he knew that the amputation could save his son's life.

Later, we would learn about Dr. Montgomery's morning visit. After examining Joe, he sat down at the nurse's station and began to type his report. The room curtain was open and he could see Joe out of the corner of his eye. As he was working, he noticed something moving, looked up and his heart sank — Joe's right arm was moving up and down — and he appeared to be having a seizure. Then he remembered that Joe was paralyzed and could not be having a seizure. He was moving his arm! He jumped up and went to Joe's bedside. Joe's arm was at his side just as it had been earlier. Had he imagined the movement? No, Joe moved his arm again.

Dr. Watson and a couple of nurses joined him and they began to put Joe through the paces, eventually discovering that he could open his eyes and look around, nod or shake his head to answer questions, and shrug both shoulders. He couldn't move his hands, fingers, or legs but his head, shoulders and upper arms were coming on-line. It was an exciting time for the doctors as they confirmed that the IVIG treatment was working!

When we arrived, we were excited to see that Joe could move his head to look at things and attempted to communicate with us by blinking his eyes (once for yes, twice for no) or shaking/nodding his head ever so slightly. We saw that he could move both arms slightly. We learned that he had responded to pain in his legs even though he still couldn't move them on his own. We were asked to watch for signs of brain and/or spinal cord damage. Joe ran a fever all day, but the doctors weren't too concerned as they thought it was probably from the IVIG.

In the evening, when Scotty came on, he gave Joe some Tylenol through his feeding tube in an attempt to bring the fever down.

When that didn't work, he ordered an Arctic Sun and put it on him. The Arctic Sun is a machine that plugs into the wall and pumps cold water into pads that wrap around the legs and body. Scotty ordered the smallest size pads and they were still big enough to swallow Joe's little body up. In a very short time, the fever started to come down and Steven & I felt comfortable enough to leave for the night. We were confident that Scotty would take good care of him, and I made sure he still had my cell phone number. It had been a very good day.

Chapter 12

Tuesday, October 10

Hospital Gets Back to Normal

Steven and I were mentally drained and slept late, hurrying to the hospital and stopping for an early lunch in the galley. It was the first time we'd eaten there, as it had been closed the entire holiday weekend. The galley was located in the basement and food was served cafeteria style. There were several stations one could go to: sandwiches, salads, ethnic food, today's special, drinks, etc. We were pleased to find a good variety of food, and healthy food too, at very reasonable prices. We each got a garden burger, French fries, drink plus 2 boxes of cereal for the next day's breakfast, all for $5.00. We were glad to have such a nice place to eat. We were also astounded to see the number of people in the building, it was as if someone had unlocked the doors and people had flooded in.

When we got to Joe's room, he was fever free and the arctic sun was turned off. He had a new nurse, an Asian lady with a nice smile who seemed very knowledgeable. We were told that we didn't have to wear the masks anymore — hallelujah — just the gowns and gloves.

Joe was awake and very alert. They had changed out his I.V. lines, removing several of them, including one at the neck that had tested positive for staph. He'd gone from 8 to 4 IVs since the last time we'd seen him. He'd also had a sponge bath and a back rub, so I was sure he felt better. He had a hand held alphabet machine and we used it to try to communicate with him. Steven held the machine close to him and I helped steady his hand with mine. He was able to point to the letters but was worn out before he could spell a full word. He was still too weak, so we put it away.

When Dr. Montgomery came in, we talked about the other cases of ADEM. We already knew that Joe was the 4th case of smallpox vaccination-induced ADEM that the military had seen in recent history. We also knew that they had learned from each case and the outcome had been better each time. He would never come out and say exactly what happened to the first three cases, but we got the distinct impression that none of them were still alive.

After he left, we started talking to Joe, telling him the story of his illness, or as much of it as we knew. He nodded his head when we told him how he'd gotten sick in Iraq, and we were sure that he remembered. He squinched his eyes when we told him he'd gone to Germany (obviously didn't know that), opened his eyes wide when we told him we'd gone to Germany too (more news), and shook his head when we told him he was at Bethesda. "Do you know where that is?" Steven asked. He shook his head no. We explained that Bethesda was near Washington D.C. and he was in a Navy hospital and his eyes opened wide again. It was a lot of news but he seemed to be understanding. I could only imagine what it would be like to go to sleep in a hospital in Iraq and wake up back home in America.

Steven began to read the stats from the machines he was hooked up to — blood pressure, oxygen content, pulse, etc. After he'd read them all, he asked Joe if he'd like to know what time it was. Joe looked at the clock on the opposite wall.

"That's funny," I said, "I didn't think he could see that clock." He turned his head and gave me a strange look.

I took my glasses off and looked at the clock, "No, I can't read it without my glasses. I'm sure he can't read it either." His eyesight was even worse than mine.

He looked at me again and squinched his eyes. "Can you see that clock?" I asked him. He nodded "yes".

"How can you see that clock when you don't have your glasses on?" I asked (like he could answer me). He gave me that same look again. Suddenly it hit me!

"Do you have your contacts in?" I asked. He nodded "yes".

Steven and I looked at each other and, together, we both said "No." Then we got down low and looked at Joe's eyes from different angles to see if we could see the lenses. I was shocked but fairly certain that I could see edges of plastic on his eyeballs. I went to get the nurse.

When Joe joined the Marine Corps he had to go to the MEP center in Kansas City three times while most recruits only go once. The first time, he scored a "0" on the ASVAB and had to sit for hours while they worked on the computer he had used. They were pretty sure it was a computer error because NOBODY had ever scored a "0". By the time they fixed it — and found that his score of 96 was the second highest of the day — it was too late for him to take the physical. A week later he went back to the MEP center but failed the physical because his eyes tested 20/800 (right at the minimum allowed). He had to go to an ophthalmologist for a more thorough exam, and then apply for a waiver. After getting the waiver, he was cleared to enlist on his 3rd trip to the MEP center. So I knew, with vision as bad as his, that there was no way he was reading the clock on the other side of the room.

Joe's nurse gave me a strange look and I knew she thought I'd lost my mind, but she brought a little flashlight with her and shined the light into his eyes. Yes, she was shocked but thought she could see contacts too, and she went to get Dr. King, the ICU doctor on duty. He was surprised to hear the story but shined a light at the side of Joe's eyes and confirmed that there were, indeed, contact lenses in his eyes. He had had those lenses in his eyes for at least 10 days! Dr. King called the ophthalmology department and within 10 minutes two people arrived to check it out. They looked in Joe's eyes and also saw the contacts. They put a drop of medicine in each eye, to help loosen the lenses, then pushed them to the corner of each eye with a Q-tip and grabbed them with their fingers.

After disposing of the lenses, they examined his eyes and decided that they were irritated, but otherwise no damage had been done. They prescribed some drops to help with the irritation, and said that he shouldn't have any lasting problems; but they were disappointed that nobody had noticed the contacts earlier. I was relieved to hear that Joe would be alright, put his glasses on him and he seemed content. I was sure that his eyes felt much better.

Soon Joe motioned for the alphabet machine, wanting to communicate with us. Again, Steven held the machine and I helped guide his hand. It was slow, which frustrated him; and at one point, he motioned for the pen I was holding in my other hand. I put it in his hand and held the paper to it, but he couldn't co-ordinate his fingers enough to write, so we went back to the machine. He would point to a letter and we would ask him if that was the letter he wanted, then he would nod or shake his head slightly. It took a long time, but he finally spelled out M-Y. Steven asked him "My. Is the first word 'my'?" Joe nodded yes. Second word. S-T-U. Steven said, "Stuff, is the second word 'stuff'?" Joe nodded yes and tried to smile, relieved that he'd gotten through to us. "You want to know what's happened to your stuff?" Steven asked. Joe nodded yes.

Steven told him that we'd gotten his backpack and what we'd found in it. He made a face. "Do you want to know about the rest of your stuff in Iraq?", Steven asked. Joe nodded yes. We told him that we didn't know but would try to find out. He rolled his eyes, that was obviously NOT the answer he was looking for. We were very pleased that he was so aware of where he was and what was going on. The doctors had told us that he could have brain damage, so that was a good sign. Soon he started showing signs of fatigue. We told him that we were going to leave for awhile so he could sleep and he nodded his head. He was tired.

We left the room about 3:00 and went to the BX, which had also been closed for the holiday. We needed to purchase a few things — more vitamins, umbrellas, heavier sweatshirts, etc. We were both happy with the progress that Joe had made that day! We called Teri and Lou, to share the good news. Lou wanted to know when Joe would be ready to come home and I had to say that I didn't know. He seemed to be getting along well at Teri's but still not understanding how sick Joe was. I also called my dad & step mom to tell them the good news. We took our purchases back to the Navy Lodge, then hurried back to the hospital. The galley was closed so we went to Subway again for another pizza.

We got back to ICU about 5:45 and, as we were putting on our isolation gowns, Joe's nurse told us that he'd had some visitors while we were gone. We were surprised to hear that and noticed that he was holding something in his hands, two coins — one from the Sgt. Major of the Marine Corps and the other from the Commandant of the Marine Corps. The highest officer and highest enlisted man in the Corps. How exciting! Joe was smiling from ear to ear — as much as he could smile with the ventilator in. It is a real honor for a Marine to meet either one of these men, and to meet them both was overwhelming. I wished I'd been there to take pictures.

Joe couldn't tell us then, but we learned later that there had been a photographer with the Sgt. Major and Commandant and they did take some pictures. We got copies of them, one of which was even signed by the Commandant.

At 6:15 the nurse asked us to leave during their shift change. It was the first time we'd been asked to leave and I took it as a sign that Joe was getting better. As we prepared to leave, we noticed that Joe looked uncomfortable. We asked the nurses to adjust his position and they went right into his room. Things seem to be going much better and we decided to do some exploring.

We'd heard that there were some computers in the visitor's lounge on the 5th floor, so we went looking for them. We found a TV, VCR, several chairs & couches, a telephone, and 4 computers in the room. We each took a computer and spent some time sending e-mails. We also made some phone calls. We went back to the lounge each day and I would send a mass e-mail to everyone in my address book, so everyone would know how Joe was doing. I could also get on my work e-mail, answer what I could, and forward other e-mails to people who could get the job done for me. I was able to read the daily bulletin and keep up with the news from school. It was good to know that there were people back home pulling for us.

Steven and I returned to ICU at 8:15 and met the new night nurse, a young, light skinned black man with a shaved head. He was very nice, but he was called away to help in another room almost immediately. While he was gone, one of Joe's medications ran out and the alarm sounded. Another nurse, who looked like Wanda Sykes, came in to turn it off. Now that the holiday was behind us, it seemed that a whole new crew was working. Joe seemed comfortable and content to watch all the action in the hallways.

We met the father of the Marine in the next room, Room 4. His son had come in from Germany on Sunday with injuries from an IED over the right side of his body. He had a shattered leg and other bones, a head injury, and the doctors were afraid that he might lose his right eye.

The ICU unit was arranged in such a way that the war wounded patients were kept separate from the retirees and dependents. The room numbers started on one end of the hall, with rooms 1 - 10 on one side and rooms 11 - 20 coming back up the other side. The war wounded patients were on the west side, rooms 1 - 5 and 16 - 20; and the other patients were on the east side, rooms 6 - 10 and 11 -15. There were two nurses' stations in the middle, so the rooms were about 30 feet away from the rooms on the opposite side. Joe was in Room 5 which was directly across the hall from Room 16. The Sharp boy, whose family we met in Germany, was in Room 17. On this day, a new patient came into Room 18, next to Sharp's room. There was a lot of activity in the room and we could hear the doctors loudly trying to wake the patient.

They would shout, "Wake up, Andrew", "Andrew, open your eyes", "Can you open your eyes for me Andrew", and finally, "Andrew, your mother is here, can you open your eyes for your mother?" Soon they put the flags on his room number — a U.S. Flag and a Marine flag. Andrew was a Marine. We saw his parents coming and going from his room each day and listened as they tried, again and again, to get Andrew to open his eyes. Joe would tell us later that he would wake up in the middle of the night, as they shouted Andrew's name.

He would lay there wishing Andrew would open his eyes so he could get some sleep!

When Joe's nurse returned, he told us that they had turned Joe's ventilator down several times that day, but each time he'd gotten distressed so they'd turned it back up. They planned to continue to try turning it down every few hours during the night, to try to wean him off it. They planned to take off the rest of the Arctic cooling blanket, continue the same medications, and check his blood sugar levels every 1 to 2 hours during the night. They had removed his Arterial lines, so they'd have to poke a finger each time they checked his blood sugar. Joe's blood sugar levels were high because of the high dose of steroids he was on, and they expected him to go back to normal when he came off the steroids. Steroids have to be gradually decreased so that would take several weeks.

As we were preparing to leave, Joe seemed stressed out, like he didn't want us to go. We weren't sure why he would be so stressed as we'd come and gone several times over the past couple of days. I felt sure that he knew we'd return but still felt guilty about leaving him. It was like his first few days of pre-school, so many years ago. I think I would have stayed the night if that had been an option. But it wasn't, and as we forced ourselves to go, I tried not to let him see me cry. Later, we would learn that he was having hallucinations from the drugs he was on — and not all of them were pleasant. When we would leave, the nurses would increase the diprivan (they also called it milk of amnesia), which helped him sleep, and the hallucinations would return.

I called Joe's friend, Andy, on the walk back to the Lodge. They had been friends since grade school and they had both, independently, decided to join the Marine Corps. Joe had once told me how surprised he was when Andy told him that he'd wanted to join for years but never told him. Of course, he hadn't told Andy that he was joining either! Andy was a year behind Joe in school, and had graduated from boot camp just 6 months earlier. He was still in training and was always anxious to hear the latest news on Joe's condition.

Once again, it was after midnight as we topped the hill near the Navy Lodge. We looked to our left and saw 4 deer laying in the meadow. It was soothing to see them laying there so calmly, just watching us as we walked by. We could barely make them out in the shadows of the trees under the street lights. They were not afraid and it calmed my nerves. I believed that it was yet another sign. We were tired and sleep came quickly.

Chapter 13

Wednesday, October 11

Movie Day

Dr. King was in Joe's room when we arrived and said that Joe had had a good night. They had been successful at turning the respirator down and planned to try removing it later in the day. Joe was also scheduled for an MRI and had already had an EKG. We met Jim, his nurse for the day. He didn't have a name badge and had written his name on a piece of masking tape and stuck it to his shirt. He had a great sense of humor and we liked him instantly. He reminded Steven of Lt. Dan, from the movie Forrest Gump, so that became his nickname for us. The respiratory therapists had been there and changed out part of the equipment that held the breathing tube in place. The new equipment didn't have straps going around his head like the old one and it looked a lot more comfortable.

When Dr. Montgomery came in he said that he'd be testing Joe's blood to figure the half-life of the gammagobulin he'd been given. We asked Jim, the nurse, if we could use the cell phone for a few minutes so Joe's dad could talk to him. Cell phones usually aren't allowed in ICU because they can interfere with some of the machines, but since none of those particular machines were being used in any nearby rooms, he let us do it. I got Lou on the phone then held it to Joe's ear so he could talk to him and it seemed to calm them both.

I noticed that Room 4 was vacant, the Marine flag was off the wall, all the furniture is out in the hall and a housekeeping crew was cleaning the room. Justin had moved upstairs. That was the big goal for the boys in ICU — to be moved up to the 5th floor — a sure sign that things were getting better!

Jim was concerned that Joe was getting bored and needed some entertainment. There was no television in the room, so he went to look for one. Soon he was back with a TV with a built-in DVD player. He'd gotten it from the Marine office and he also brought some DVDs. He showed them all to Joe then told him to nod his head when he got to the one he wanted to see, and showed them to him again. Joe picked "Dracula". I chuckled because he is a HUGE vampire and zombie fan. We all sat down to watch and 30 minutes later Joe was sound asleep.

Steven & I went to the galley for lunch while Joe was sleeping and he called Sgt. Nichols to set up his flight home. His boss was scheduled to go in for surgery so he had to get back to work soon. I wished he could stay longer, but he would be leaving on his birthday, October 15. When we got back to ICU, Dracula was over and Joe was still sleeping.

Dr. Watson, the neurologist, and one of his interns came in to examine Joe, but they couldn't get him to wake up. They finally decided to wait another day to do a more thorough exam.

We had discovered that we had to plan our meals well in advance at Bethesda. While there were several eating places in the hospital building, most of them were closed before dinner time. The galley closed at 1 pm and the food court, which had a nice variety of restaurants, including Taco Bell, Portabellas, Pizza Hut, a sandwich shop, and Chinese food, closed at 3 pm. That left Subway, vending machines, or a short walk to McDonald's as dinner choices. We had gotten into the habit of getting our food early and microwaving it for dinner. While Joe was asleep, we made our "dinner run" and took the food to the Lodge; it was just starting to drizzle when we got there.

My dad called while we were there, they were at my house in Springfield and were having trouble getting in. I knew that the front door was locked, but I had left a spare key on the back porch, just in case. I had also unlocked the back storm door and told Lou to leave it unlocked but, he had apparently gone behind me and locked it anyway! Dad had gotten in by removing the frame of the storm door; then using the key I'd left to open the main door. They had gotten the mail from our neighbors, sorted it out, threw the junk mail away, took the bills out and left the rest on the table for me. We had made a plan for them to pay the bills so I wouldn't have my utilities cut off or be charged late fees, then I would reimburse them when I got home. They had talked to my neighbor Tom, who mowed my lawn yesterday. I have the best neighbors. Grace watered my house plants and threw out the spoiled food in the refrigerator. They were just locking the house and heading back to their home in Clinton (about 85 miles away), it was good to know that they were taking care of things at home.

When Steven & I got back to the hospital, we found Joe awake and watching "The Lord of the Rings". We stayed with him until 6:30, when the nurses asked us to leave during their shift change. We put "Back to the Future" in the DVD player, went to the Lodge for dinner, and returned to the hospital at 8:30. I enjoyed all the walking and hoped it might even help me with my weight loss efforts. When we got back to the hospital, Joe had grown tired of movies and was having some breathing problems. We turned off the TV and had the nurse clean the congestion out of his ventilator tube (which he hated), and then he went right to sleep. Steven & I went back to the Lodge, watched the news and went to sleep too. I guess we were all tired.

Chapter 14

Thursday, October 12
Coming off the Ventilator

When Steven & I got to the hospital, Dr. King was waiting to talk to us. They had turned the ventilator down in the early morning hours and Joe had been breathing on his own for about five hours! He had been on the ventilator for a total of 11 days and they were anxious to get him off it before he developed pneumonia or vocal cord problems. We were able to spend about 10 minutes with him before the portable x-ray machine arrived and they asked us to step out of the room. We took the opportunity to leave the floor, using our cell phones to call everyone at home with the good news. The x-ray looked good and Steven and I watched as they took out the ventilator tube. It was quick, but hard to watch, with Joe gagging as it came out. I looked at the clock; it was 11:15 a.m.

The respiratory therapists put an oxygen mask on Joe and connected it to a nebulizer, telling us that they would give him medication every few hours, to help with his chest congestion. He was told to cough as much as possible to loosen the congestion in his lungs, and keep him from developing pneumonia.

Joe wanted to talk, but the ventilator tube had irritated his voice box and he was unable to speak above a whisper. We had to lean over, putting our ears near his mouth to hear him. We were still watching for signs of brain damage and wanted him to talk so we could test his short term memory, long term memory, problem solving skills, etc. At one point, I was prodding him to tell me something that should have been easy for him, but he wouldn't answer me. He gave me his 'do you think I'm stupid?' look and I pushed him again to answer me. "Oh", I said "is that one too hard for you?"

He looked me in the eye and whispered as forcefully as he could, "Fuck you!"

I burst out laughing, greatly relieved, and instantly knew that his brain was fine. Steven was puzzled and asked "What? What did he say?"

It took me a minute to compose myself long enough to tell him what Joe had just said.. Then I said "There's nothing wrong with his mind, he's just fine!"

I realize that most parents would be horrified to hear such words from their child, but it was music to my ears! While I tell the students at my school that they shouldn't use the word, I have never been insulted by it. Joe would know that he could answer me in that way only if his brain was normal, so I knew that his brain was fine, even if his body wasn't. I was ecstatic!

After all that talking (whispering), Joe was thirsty and asking for water but the doctors were afraid he might choke on it. They let us swab his mouth with a wet toothbrush-like sponge and the moisture seemed to satisfy him. He was tired and began to doze off, so Steven

& I left so he could sleep. We went to the galley for lunch, then to the BX to buy a battery charger for Joe's IPOD.

When we got back to Joe's room he was awake and watching movies again. We plugged his IPOD into the charger and watched movies with him until they kicked us out for shift change. He was relaxed and enjoyed being free of the ventilator. After dinner, we returned to his room and found that he was very alert and full of energy. The nurses had told us that he'd probably be awake for a long time when they took him off the ventilator (and the medicines that went along with it) and they were right. He spent the next several hours telling us stories. We gave him ice chips when his throat got sore. Since he couldn't talk above a whisper, Steven would lean over close enough to hear him, and then repeat the stories to me so I could write them down. These are the stories he told us, in his own words, many of them were hallucinations roughly based on what was going on around him:

Hallucination #1 — When I first woke up, I was in a hole that had sticks coming out of the sides. People were all around and someone said "The Shaman wants to see you". All I could think about was the shaman in Pirates of the Caribbean II, so I thought "what's a shaman and what am I doing here?" Then I had to get an MRI, it was a weird MRI, all trippy like an acid trip. Mom was saying "you're going to be alright", but she was in a Japanese guy's way and he was just trying to get out of the hole. I had a big tube in my mouth and mom said "don't touch it." I was going to get BMI test and someone covered me in oil. Steven accidentally pulled the tube out of my nose. He asked if it was alright and they said "we'll just give him another one". After the test I had to go down 2 stories to get dunked in water and there were a bunch of munchkins there. It started to snow around the water tank. We went back upstairs and talked to the Japanese guy (he saw us coming and jumped back into the hole so he could get a good shot). Mom put her head in the hole, blocking it so the Japanese guy couldn't get out. The guy was trapped in the hole. I went to sleep; they did another MRI, then let me rest.

Hallucination #2 — On day two there was a crazy nurse, who wasn't supposed to be working, she took $100,000, gave me cortisone shots, and tried to kill me. Steve was hiding under the bed with a video camera and had filmed it all. We went to a room, it was a cool room, we messed up the stage and the guy there called Steve a sick-a-fant. Steve tried to get me to go with him but I couldn't move; when Steve didn't believe me, I said "I physically can't move." The stage was covered with shoes, and the walls were next to people's rooms, so when they moved the stage, it pissed everyone off. Steve pleaded with me for about 30 minutes to go, and when the nurse saw him on the floor, she said "what the hell?" I gave her a weird look. When the doctor came into room, the nurse was cleaning up poop, and the doctor asked "is everything OK?" The nurse said "I'm just cleaning up," the doctor saw Steve on floor but said OK and left. I lay there a long time.

Hallucination #3 — I was going to be NJPed (punished by an officer) because I'd been drinking. Mom showed up and they tried to freeze the alcohol by putting something cold on my chest. But I hadn't been drinking; I had only had a Pepsi. I didn't know the general would be there and I was throwing up. They said I still had .8 blood alcohol level. They thought I was drunk and kept trying to do the test. The Lt. General said he was going to knock me down to private, and then they tried to freeze it out again. Two days later I took the test again, got orders but it was 14 days before I had to leave for Iraq so they couldn't do anything to me. So I got away with it. There were 150 guys there that I'd just met and the Lt. General came on intercom and said that he wanted everyone to know that the career of LCpl Lopez was over and everyone must work to be sure things like that didn't happen again. Then he talked about himself. There was a delusional guy who said he'd just flown in from Normandy, when he got shot down and they all told him he was 60 years too late for that. There was a kid he called Lucky because he had no legs and they gave him electronic legs. I was pissed off about the drinking ordeal — it was the first time I'd almost gotten NJPed. Mom showed up and was mad because they weren't taking care of me. I sat there without blood for about 3 hours while waiting to see if they wanted to NJP me. I felt like I was about to pass out.

Hallucination #4 — The next day (Monday) they wanted to give me shots in the butt but they had a real gun. It was scary. Steve & Mom left during this because Sheri (mom's sister) and her six kids came over. They all came back in the middle of the night. Christopher (the oldest kid) was acting up so they shot him in the head with a carbon cannon. They were trying to get inside. They had to use the base defenses to keep them away. They were yelling "let me in". That night we filled out restriction papers in blood so Sheri couldn't come around. The doctor called them an embarrassment because they were making such asses of themselves.

Hallucination #5 — There were kids running around the hospital selling air & water, it was some kind of a fund raising project.

Hallucination #6 — My bed had a big dog underneath it that would try to get up, shaking the bed. I was afraid the dog would bite somebody. One of the nurses got a tranquilizer gun and tried to shoot the dog, but she shot me instead. She hit me with both tranquilizer darts.

Hallucination #7 — On Tuesday, there was a crazy nurse with 2 million dollars in the other ICU room. I was supposed to go out that morning but they gave me a physical and said they would have to make me walk. They shot the big dog that was under my bed. The crazy nurse took care of me that night, gave me "quick clot" which closes up the pores if you're shot but can kill you if you don't need it. I said "I don't need this," she said "You'll be alright" and gave me more — 800 cc — I knew you would get ulcers if you had too much, then they gave me fluids, really pumped it into me. She kept doing crazy things like that. Then Steven & mom finally got there. Crazy nurse missed 3 flights. She didn't even know what hemoglobin was. The doctor said "find me a bag for him" and the nurse searched for about an hour to find out what hemoglobin was. She didn't know what sterilization was and when Steven & mom got there, they had the dog under the bed, had shot me in the face with tranquilizer, and I passed out.

Hallucination #8 — The next day I woke up and the doctors did an exam to check on stomach ulcers, they thought it might have something to do with the quick clot. After about 3 hours, they started talking to crazy nurse about her not being able to practice medicine anymore. Five hours later we filled out forms on malpractice, the settlement came out to 2 million dollars, they kept messing up forms but finally got it filled out and Steven & I went to the Millionaire's Club to watch over the $100,000 we had there. Crazy lady, her 2 kids and 1 other kid were there talking about trying to kill us by running us off the road and they thought they would keep all our money. Steve kept kicking his chair, she said I would have to leave if she came in, the orderly threw ink, I filed police report, and they went to jail. Sheri and her kids came to do voice-overs for the police report.

Hallucination #9 — The walls seemed to move and there were psychedelic colors on them, like someone had painted them with wildly colored paint that moved strangely. A Marine came into the room with a gun, obviously wanting to shoot me. I lay very still; he didn't see me and moved on down the hall looking for me. After he left, there were bears that seemed to walk through the walls, danced around my room, then faded back into the walls.

Some of his stories were very strange, and at one point, Joe looked at me and said "You know, I left Fallujah in a body bag." I was amazed and wondered if it was another hallucination. Perhaps they had wrapped him tightly in a blanket. "No, it was a body bag. They even cut a hole in it for my head. They said it was for warmth." Steven & I just looked at each other, not sure what to think!

Steven & I were amazed at Joe's stories. Some of them seemed to go along with actual events but others seemed to be pure hallucinations. He thought that Steven had hidden a video camera with video of some of the things that had happened in his hallucinations, and we had to convince him that there was no video camera. We spent hours listening to the stories and telling him what had really happened.

Joe finally started getting tired so we gave him his, now charged up, IPOD. As he joyfully but tediously flipped through the songs, with fingers that barely worked, I wondered what he would listen to first. He finally found what he was looking for and I asked, "What are you going to listen to?" He smiled and said "Big Smith". Big Smith is a hillbilly band from Springfield, and one of our favorite local bands. They had been with him all the way to Iraq and back, a piece of home. I left him enjoying one of our favorite songs, "Three Speed, Twelve Inch Oscillating Fan". It was another sign that his brain was functioning normally and as Steven and I walked up the hill toward the Navy Lodge our elation turned to exhaustion.

CHAPTER 15

Friday, October 13

Glen's Visit

When we arrived in ICU, we saw Mrs. George, one of the first nurses to care for Joe. She had been off work for a week and had seen Joe for the first time that morning. She was amazed at how good he looked and actually had tears in her eyes when she talked to us. Being an ICU nurse must be a tough job.

Around noon the respiratory therapists came in and gave Joe a breathing treatment; followed by Ms. Huet, a speech pathologist, who examined his throat; then Dr. Sebeny, an infectious disease specialist.

Early in the afternoon my friend, Glen, arrived.. We had known each other since high school and corresponded by e-mail, but hadn't actually seen each other since college. He was currently living near D.C., worked in the city, and rode the metro past BNMC each day. It was good to see him after so many years and we had a nice visit. He enjoyed talking to Steven, the years seemed to melt away, and soon it was as if we'd just seen each other a few days earlier. We were able to visit for a couple of hours before it was time for him to catch the metro home.

While we were visiting, they took Joe for a swallow test. Steven went with him and enjoyed watching the x-ray machine as the fluid traveled down Joe's esophagus. Joe did fairly well, but didn't totally pass. The doctors decided that he would only be able to eat and drink thick items. I made a quick call to tell Lou the good news then hurried back for Joe's first taste of food, lemon jello, which he enjoyed immensely. The respiratory therapists returned for another breathing treatment & breathing exercises, followed by Dr. Montgomery. He didn't stay long but said that Joe was doing well. Soon after he left Joe got to eat orange jello, then it was time for us to leave during shift change. Scotty would be his overnight nurse.

Steve & I went to our second family dinner in the executive dining room; arriving late, but welcomed with open arms. The food was excellent, once again, and there were more families than at the last meal. When we returned to ICU around 8:00 pm, Scotty was checking Joe's insulin level and Joe watching a John Wayne movie. There was a woman screaming at the nurses in the civilian part of ICU, something about her relative not getting proper care. She went on and on, swearing and yelling at the nurses. It was pretty pathetic. Her tantrum was much, much worse than the one I had had a few days earlier! By 8:30, Joe was asleep so we walked back to the Lodge. I saw the woman who had been ranting at the nurses, as we passed by the room. She was a middle aged black woman and was sitting in a chair next to an older gentleman in the bed; I thought that he was probably her father.

Chapter 16

Saturday, October 14

Sitting up and Getting a Shave

When we arrived at the hospital, Dr. Bennett told us that he was satisfied with Joe's progress. He was scheduled for an MRI at noon, so Steven & I followed his bed as far as we could then sat in the MRI waiting room and watched baseball on TV.

After the MRI, Joe got his first taste of real food for lunch. Steven and I fed him tomato soup, potato soup, banana pudding, strawberry ice cream and milk, all thick liquids, and he ate a little of each item. He had barely finished eating when the respiratory therapists arrived for another breathing treatment, he didn't like them, but it was better than being on the ventilator. Steven & I went to Subway for our own lunch, helping Joe with his IPOD before we left. He liked listening to it while he slept, and using the ear buds blocked out the hospital noise.

When we got back to Joe's room, he was sitting up in a recliner-type chair with an oxygen mask on. The nurse told us that he'd had some trouble breathing and she thought it was probably from the congestion. Sitting more up-right seemed to help with his breathing. Soon it was dinner time (more tomato soup, chocolate pudding, an energy drink and vanilla ice cream), followed by another breathing treatment.

We decided that Joe needed some sprucing up, so Steven got a razor and shaving cream and gave him a shave and then I washed his hair. It seemed to make him feel better. All too soon, the respiratory therapists were back again for another breathing treatment. He was getting a lot of treatments as one lung had started collapsing a little on bottom. They planned to put a mask on him that night while he was sleeping to help open up his lungs.

Around 8:00, Scotty lifted Joe from the chair to his bed and discovered that his catheter was leaking. He would have to put in a larger one, but he promised to numb things up first. Steven & I took a walk and made phone calls while they were doing it, neither of us wanted to stay for that procedure. Soon after Joe was settled back in bed, Dr. T came in. He said that Joe was surprising everyone with his progress. His case was so very rare and he'd made such great progress, he thought that doctors would be writing about him in medical journals some day and using what they had learned from him to help others with his condition.

"Good thing you didn't let him bleed to death," I thought!

Scotty was also in a talkative mood and spent quite awhile telling Joe what he might expect to happen with the military: possible medical discharge, veteran's benefits he could qualify for, war zone benefits, etc. One thing he stressed was the importance of getting a copy of his medical records. We would find, as time went on, that everybody stressed the importance of having your own copy. Joe started getting sleepy around 9:00 so we gave him his IPOD, and Steven & I walked to the Lodge. Steven would be leaving the next day and he was worried about me walking back and forth alone, after dark. He tried to convince me that I needed to ask the Marine liaisons to drive me. I told him I'd think about it but, deep down, I knew that I wouldn't; I just liked the walk.

Chapter 17

Sunday, October 15

Steven's Birthday and His Last Day

When I woke up, I knew it would be a sad day. Steven had to be back at work on Monday, so he had to catch a plane that afternoon. The Marines had arranged for his flight home and he finished packing his suitcase before our walk to the hospital. He planned to leave it in Joe's room until time to go. We stopped at the Marine Liaison office on the first floor to make sure there would be a driver to take him to the airport. He chuckled at the thought of having been to Washington D.C. twice, never leaving the hotel where his meetings were the first time and never leaving the base this time. He commented that someday he'd like to see the sights.

When we got to ICU, Joe had finished breakfast and Dr. Fu, the neurologist of the day, had just finished examining him. He hadn't slept well with the breathing mask on. The machine was very loud, the way it pushed the air into his lungs was irritating and he had finally convinced the nurses to take it off. Joe's upper body had been getting stronger every day. He was able to move his arms far enough to scratch his nose with either hand, and had been exercising his left hand so he could give a thumbs up to his visitors. He had some sensation in his legs from time to time but still no movement there. He had been seen by Dr. Miller earlier in the morning. Dr. Miller was a neurologist who had had Guillain-Barre 24 years earlier and still walked with an arm crutch. He told Joe that he still had small improvements from time to time, even after 24 years! It was encouraging!

Sheri called to tell me that there was trouble with Lou. He wasn't doing well and she was also worried about Teri. Teri had stopped taking her medicine so she would be awake when Lou got up to wander around during the night. She had found him outside a couple of nights ago and she was afraid he'd wander off and get lost. Teri had her own medical issues, as she had been diagnosed with M.S. about 2 years earlier, and we all worried about her. She had always been very healthy and active and it had been a real challenge for her to have to admit that she was not well. She had quit working about 6 months earlier and her husband had passed away about a month before Joe got sick. Teri had 3 kids, 2 of them in high school, that she was raising by herself. Her life had really changed and I knew that having Lou living there had been hard for her. I decided that it was time to make arrangements to move him. Later, I would learn that Sheri hadn't told me everything; things were a lot worse than I knew.

I tried to call the memory clinic, where Lou was treated for Alzheimer's, but only got an answering machine. I called Dr. Del Rosa's office, his general practitioner, and got the nurse on call. She agreed to have the doctor call Sheri and give her some recommendations.

I got back to Joe's room in time for his breathing treatment, and a visit from Dr. Foote. The nurse changed the Foley bag and checked

Joe's blood sugar. Soon it was time for lunch: more soup, pudding, and protein drink.

Steven & I ate lunch at Subway, and then went back to Joe's room. He hated to leave while Joe was still in ICU, and waited till the last minute to tell him goodbye. I walked with him to the 1st floor Marine liaison office, and then watched as he got into the van and drove away. The tears flowed again; it had been such a blessing to have him there. Now I would have to make all the decisions on my own, for Joe and also for Lou, and there would be some tough decisions to be made in the next few days and weeks. I spent some time alone before going back to Joe's room. I didn't want him to see me cry, I didn't want him to worry about me, and he needed all his strength for himself.

The evening was pretty uneventful; Joe had his dinner (same food as lunch) and another breathing treatment. We watched a movie and he started getting sleepy. I think we were both sad that Steven was gone and neither of us wanted to burden the other with our sadness. Around 9:00, he was sleepy and asked for his IPOD, and I left for the Lodge. I thought for a minute about asking for a ride, but only for a minute, it was dark but I was on a Navy base, for Pete's sake. I felt safe and, besides, the walk would give me a chance to think, to unwind, and maybe make a phone call. There was a message from Steven, he had made it home.

Chapter 18

Monday, October 16

I Am Alone

I woke up alone and tried to remember the last time that had happened. I couldn't remember back that far. It seemed that I'd always had someone with me: husband, kids, brothers & sisters, parents. Had I ever been alone? I was sure I must have been, but I couldn't remember. I had to smile, I really couldn't remember. I ate a bowl of cereal in my room, did the laundry, and made telephone calls to Missouri. I needed to get Lou into a nursing home and it had to be in Missouri. Since his health insurance didn't cover nursing homes, I would have to apply for Medicaid or pay for it myself — and since the cost would be more than I brought home each month, it would have to be Medicaid. I'd have to handle it by phone calls and faxes and I would find that everyone was considerate of my situation and most helpful. People are good.

When I got to Joe's room, he was awake and no longer on oxygen. Soon the nurse came in and disconnected his last IV. They left the IV needle in his arm, just in case they needed it again, but he was finally disconnected from all those tubes! Dr. Cirivellos told me that they planned to move him to the 5th floor soon. The fifth floor was where all the military patients went, either to the surgical side or the medical side, depending on their condition. Getting out of ICU would be HUGE for Joe!

Soon it was time for another breathing treatment, followed by Dr. Fu and the neurology team. She said they would be doing a test on his lungs which would determine when he would be moved out of ICU.

After helping Joe eat his lunch, I went to the galley to eat my own lunch and make more phone calls about Lou. I couldn't get any information from his Springfield doctors but I did get through to Teri. Lou had, once again, been up all night and was now asleep, naked, on the bedroom floor. I was feeling guilty that Teri had to deal with Lou, as I hurried back to Joe's room.

While I was gone, Joe had a chest x-ray and breathing test. Soon Dr. Miller and the neurology team came in and examined him.

After they left, I went back to work on Lou's situation, picking up a Medicaid application from the fax machine, filling it out and faxing it to the nursing home in Springfield that the Memory Clinic had located. I talked to Teri several times, at first she couldn't wake Lou and had decided to let him sleep as long as possible. Then Sheri and her husband, Mike, arrived and also tried to wake him. Sheri had once worked at a nursing home and knew how to handle Alzheimer's patients.

When I got back to ICU, the occupational therapist had been to see Joe and told him that she would bring him a fork and spoon with large, rubber handles so he could start feeding himself. I was sure he would like the freedom of that. Since I couldn't use my cell phone in

ICU, I had turned it to vibrate so I wouldn't miss any calls about Lou. Soon it started to vibrate and I left the room to make a call.

It was the nursing home and they were faxing more papers for me to fill out. I called Teri and she told me that they had finally gotten Lou in the car and she & Sheri were driving toward Springfield with him. He had fallen in the driveway and skinned up his knees on the way to the car. That was ironic because Joe had skinned up knees too. He had skinned his knees that last night in Iraq, as his legs were going numb and he was unable to urinate, he'd pulled himself outside to the porta-john several times, and now had scabs on both knees.

Teri agreed to call me when they got Lou to the nursing home. I knew it would be hard for them. Joe's dinner arrived just as I got back to his room and I helped him eat his tomato soup, protein shake, chocolate pudding, chocolate ice cream and milk. He must have been hungry because he ate everything — it was good to see his appetite coming back. Soon it was time for another breathing treatment, then shift change, and time for me to go.

I stopped by the Liaison Office and picked up the fax from the nursing home. I walked to the Lodge, warmed up a TV dinner in the microwave and filled out the papers while I ate. Steven called and I filled him in on what had been happening all day. It sure was lonely without him. I called Teri as I walked back to the hospital and she told me that they were just leaving the nursing home. It had been hard for them to leave Lou, but it was done. Soon, Lou wouldn't even remember the drive back to Springfield; he was getting so much worse. I stopped at the Liaison office and faxed the papers back to the nursing home.

While in the Liaison office, I met Andrew's parents, and they told me that he still hadn't opened his eyes for them. They seemed like nice people and we would become friends as the weeks passed.

I hurried back to Joe's room, worried about having been gone over 2 hours, but he was fine and listening to his IPOD. He wanted to see a movie, so I put in Independence Day. My cell phone went off, it was Sheri, and I left the room to call her back. They were just leaving my house for the trip back to Tulsa. I went back to Joe's room and finished watching the movie with him. He had been very quiet all day. I decided that he was missing Steven too, and although I hadn't told him everything that was happening back home, he knew that his dad was in bad shape. I think he was afraid to ask for details and I was glad that he was saving his energy. When the movie ended, I gave him his IPOD and he went right to sleep.

It was 10:30 pm but I wanted to send some e-mails and went to the computer room, which was empty. It was good to know that Lou was in a safe place with people who could take care of him — and I was relieved that Teri wouldn't have to worry with him anymore. I would have felt so bad if she had made herself sick. She just wasn't well enough to deal with him. I had sent some e-mails to people in Springfield who knew something about the nursing homes there and was glad to get some positive responses about the one where we'd placed Lou. I felt a little guilty about him being there, thinking that, perhaps, I should go home, but I knew I couldn't leave Joe. Given the choice, I felt that I could do more good where I was.

It was after midnight when I finally left the computer room and started toward the Navy Lodge. As I passed the Marine Liaison office, I thought of Steven and how he wanted me to ask for a ride. It was too late, the office closed at midnight, and so I stepped out the door and into the darkness. The streets were empty except for a security vehicle that passed me just as I reached the street. Seeing him made me feel more at ease, and as I got to the top of the hill where we'd seen the deer a few days earlier, I saw the same car. He was sitting in a parking lot nearby, but pulled out on the road, going back toward the hospital after I passed him. That was nice. He was keeping an eye out for me. I felt secure. I got to the Lodge and fell into bed. I was really tired and sleep came swiftly.

Chapter 19

Tuesday, October 17

Out of ICU!!

I overslept and felt guilty as I left the Lodge at 10 am, walking quickly to the hospital. I was anxious to see Joe and was pleased to find that he was awake and cheerful but noticed that the VenaFlow air pumpers were turned off. These "pumpers" as I had come to call them, wrapped around his calves and hooked up to an electric machine that pumped the air in to inflate, then pulled the air out to deflate. The doctors had explained that it would help with the circulation in his lower legs and lessen the danger of blood clots. He had also been wearing hard plastic "boots" on his feet which kept his feet at 90 degree angles to his legs. The doctors said wearing the boots would keep his tendons and muscles stretched out so walking would be easier if and when the time came. While the air was turned off, I took the "pumpers" and boots off and messaged Joe's feet and calves, even though he had no feeling there. His breakfast tray was still there and I saw that he'd had grits, protein shake, pudding and

Ensure for breakfast. I thought "he'll sure be glad when some real food comes his way!"

I had barely gotten the pumpers and boots back on when things got busy. The respiratory therapists came in for a breathing treatment; followed by a hospital chaplain, infectious disease doctors (they talked about moving him to the 5th floor), speech therapist (still wants an ENT doctor to look at Joe's vocal cords) and Dr. Fu. It was like a parade, one person after another, such a flurry of activity! Dr. Fu's visit was cut short by the arrival of lunch — more delicious soup, ice cream, protein shake, pudding and Ensure. I added thickener to all the thin liquids and helped him eat. He was just happy to have food!

Joe finished his lunch just in time for me to rush to the galley for my lunch. It was almost 1 pm and I was one of the last ones in the door before they shut and locked it. I was glad I had made it because they had vegetarian fajitas and they were really good! I think I enjoyed it even more after seeing what Joe had to eat! While I was out, I called the rehab center to check on Lou, called Teri to see how she was doing, and also my dad. Then I stopped in the computer room to check my e-mail.

When I got back to Joe's room, they were getting him ready for the move to the 5th floor! We were both SO EXCITED, but it was also a scary time. There were fewer nurses on the 5th floor, so Joe would get less attention from them, which meant that I would need to spend even more time at the hospital, at least for the first few days.

Three nurses wheeled his bed out the back door of ICU, into the service elevator, and up to the 5th floor. He tried to give a thumbs up but couldn't quite make his thumb straight. He was taken to Room 4 on the medical unit, called 5 Center, where we were met by a corpsman, nurse and intern. Joe kept the same bed which they placed next to the window. It had a nice view of the tower. There was another bed in the room but it was empty, Joe would enjoy the quiet. His room was near the main elevators and just two doors down from the computer room where I had been going to check my e-mails. Across the hall was the employee locker room and the 5th Floor Marine Liaison office. It was a good location and Joe seemed to like it.

Joe's dinner seemed to be a bit more interesting than his ICU meals; instead of soup and pudding they brought him rice, mixed vegetables, cottage cheese and bread - real food! He seemed to like the variety but didn't eat a lot as he was tired from all the activity. The doctor on duty came by to see him, and then he settled in for a nap. I took the opportunity to walk to the Navy Lodge and eat my own dinner.

I was gone for nearly two hours and was surprised to see that the Vena Cuffs (pumpers) were still not hooked up when I returned. The doctors had been very concerned about blood clots, and I asked the nurse to get them turned on as soon as possible. She hadn't noticed that they weren't working and hooked them up right away. She also brought Joe some juice, which he enjoyed. The alarm on the Vena Cuffs went off again and again and for the next two hours, and the nurse and I were unable to find the problem. She finally gave up and went to look for another machine.

There were no cell phone restrictions on the fifth floor and I was able to answer mine whenever it rang. The nursing home called and Lou's nurse asked me if I could talk to him. It was the first time I'd talked to him since he'd been in the nursing home and I wasn't sure what to expect.

Lou talked about how his business trip was going and told me that he hoped to be finished and able to come home in another day or two. He thought he was still working for Thrifty Rent-a-Car and was somewhere auditing a licensee's books, which was something he had done when we first met, back in the early 80s. I went along with the story and tried to make him feel at ease. When I told him that Joe was feeling better and had been moved to another room, he was surprised to hear that he was sick. He believed that Joe & I were at home and he was staying in a hotel in another town. After about 10 minutes, he promised to call the next day and hung up. I was relieved to know that he was content and doing well.

Soon the nurse came in with a sleeping pill and laxative for Joe. It was much quieter in his new room and he began to doze off. I made sure he was comfortable, gave him his IPOD, turned out the lights and left for the Navy Lodge. It had been an exciting day.

Chapter 20

Wednesday, October 18

Settling in on the Fifth Floor

Joe spent the first week establishing a routine in his new room. We met the new doctors, nurses and corpsmen and each day was a flurry of activities. He was assigned to the Red Team and they checked on him twice a day. Student nurses came from the local college once a week, volunteers came by with magazines, occupational therapists and dieticians came in every day, physical therapists and respiratory therapists worked with him twice a day. He got a fat-handled fork and spoon and started learning to feed himself; and I was shown the pantry, where I could get ice and juice, and keep food in the refrigerator. Each day he got more "real food" and got better at feeding himself. We met Lt. Marino, the head of nursing, and he requested a chair so Joe could get out of bed from time to time.

The neurologists continued to say bad things about IVIG, and I continued to ignore them. The Red Team consisted of doctors who were doing their residency or internship at Bethesda and they were all intrigued by Joe as none of them had ever seen anyone with his illness before. The doctors reduced the steroids Joe was taking every few days, and monitored his blood sugar level before each meal. He would need an insulin shot after most of his meals while they were lowering the steroids.

Joe started receiving visitors and he got a coin from a member of the Marine League on his first day.

There were some issues, and by dinnertime that first day, I had confronted the lead doctor on the Red Team about the broken Vena Cuff machine and also the head nurse, as Joe hadn't been bathed all day, even though the supplies had been in his room since morning. Within an hour, both issues had been resolved. It was obvious that everyone on the 5th floor was overworked.

Joe's got a roommate that first evening, the peace and quiet had been short lived. His name was Brian, he was a Marine Lieutenant from the Quantico, Virginia base and he had been burned during a training exercise. They brought him in a wheelchair and he seemed to be in good spirits. We would learn that he had 2nd and 3rd degree burns on his right thigh and leg, and the emergency room doctors had just pumped him full of pain killers. He wasn't feeling any pain when he got to Room 4. Brian's wife had recently given birth to their first child, born prematurely, but almost up to the 5 pounds that he had to weigh to be discharged. He seemed to be a nice guy, not much older than Joe, and he'd been in the Marine Corps for about the same length of time. He showed us the burn on his leg — it covered most of his right thigh all the way down to his knee. He laughed when I asked him how fast he'd gotten his pants off — "pretty damn fast!" As the days went by and the pain medication wore off, his leg hurt more and more. The pain killers seemed to wear off faster each time they gave it to him, like he was building up a tolerance to it. The doctors had asked his wife to visit the baby in the infant ICU before coming to see Brian, so she wouldn't transmit germs to the NICU from the 5th floor, many of them brought back from foreign countries. So she would come to visit him each day, after seeing their baby.

Chapter 21

Thursday, October 19

Out of Room & Confrontation with Doctor

The nurses brought in a strange looking bed/chair for Joe. It was bright pink and I smiled, thinking how the Marines must love the color. The nurse would lay it down like a bed, and then crank it up until it was the same height as the bed. Next she would turn another crank which would slide a clear piece of plastic onto the bed and underneath the patient. When the patient was fully on the plastic, the nurse would turn the crank in the opposite direction and the patient would be moved off the bed onto the chair. The nurse would strap the patient to the chair, turn the first crank to lower the chair, put the arms up, and turn another crank that would raise the top portion until the patient was in a sitting position. The whole operation took about 20 minutes, but when the patient was finally in the seated position, the chair could be pushed around somewhat like a wheelchair. I say "somewhat" because the thing was VERY heavy and awkward — and steered like a Mac truck. It was good for the nurses, as they didn't have to lift the patient and we were told that it had dramatically reduced back injuries.

Since I am such an adventurer, I decided to take Joe for a stroll. "Have a nice time," the nurses said, as they smiled and waved — knowing that I would need three boys and a mule to help push the thing. We made our way, in a zigzag fashion, toward the elevators. Joe didn't care, he was out of his room for the first time in almost 3 weeks and he was so excited to have the freedom. Somehow, I managed to get him into the elevator and down to the lobby on the first floor. The lobby was pretty impressive and I acted as Joe's personal guide. There was a long line of windows that looked out over a courtyard between the buildings and, standing in front of the windows was a long line of flags, one for each state. In the center of the room, directly in front of the entry doors, there was a life-size statue of a Navy medic pulling an injured Marine to safety. It is gold in color and immediately conveyed the relationship between the two branches. I took a picture of Joe next to the statue, just as I'd seen so many others doing as I came and went from the hospital. The weather was nice, so we went out the electric doors to the circle drive and sat for awhile. Joe was happy to be breathing some fresh air but soon began to tire, so we worked our way, in zigzag style, back to the elevator and into the computer room. I acted as his secretary as he read his e-mails and I typed his replies. It was good therapy for him to see how many people were thinking about him.

Later that day, while I was out of the room, the neurology team came in. They told Joe that they wouldn't be doing another MRI or IVIG treatment and the neurologist in charge said that he probably would never get any better. He recommended that Joe get started with rehab so he could learn to live with his disability. I was livid and again had words with the Red Team leader!

First One Home

Still upset, I marched into Lt. Col. Workman's office, the Marine Liaison for the patients on the 5th floor. I said "This is MY son but he is also one of YOUR Marines and you need to get on top of this. I will not tolerate this negativity and you better not tolerate it either." Joe had only been out of ICU for two days and it was much too early to be giving up. The Lt. Colonel immediately called the head of the neurology department, who visited me later in Joe's room. It was the last time the neurologists said anything negative to Joe, and my reputation had been set.

My dad & step-mom went to see Lou in the nursing home and he was able to recognize them. He was wearing a bracelet so an alarm would sound if he got out of the building and he told them about the job he was doing (still seemed to be living in the 80s). He didn't seem to know where I was or that Joe was sick. When I called the counselor at the nursing home, he said that Lou was doing well, bonding with some of the other men; sitting and talking with them for hours at a time. He seemed to be doing well.

I saw Dr. Montgomery in the hall outside Joe's room and began talking to him there. The head of the Red Team, Dr. Fung, joined us and the two doctors started talking. Dr. Montgomery explained to him that they would be giving the same amount of IVIG over the same period of time as the last treatment. He told him what to watch for during the IVIG treatment, both the minor and major reactions. He gave Dr. Fung specific instructions as to if and when he should be called. I was interested to hear that Joe's IG level had been 500 on admission, up to 3000 after the first treatment, 2000 last week and 1200 that day. He gave Dr. Fung an impromptu quiz about IG levels, what is considered to be normal, low, dangerously low, etc. and I smiled as I watched him trying to come up with the answers. I was watching the master teacher give instruction to a pupil and I thought, again, that Dr. Montgomery would make a great teacher.

Joe was taken for an MRI that evening. It took two hours and I waited in the MRI waiting room, watching a football game and reading a newspaper. Joe was sleeping when they wheeled his bed out, woke up briefly when he got back to his room, then went right back to sleep. It had been his busiest day yet, and once again, I was exhausted as I walked up the hill toward the Navy Lodge.

Chapter 22

Friday, October 20

IVIG Treatment & Roommate Drama

The day began quietly enough as we prepared for another IVIG treatment. Dr. Montgomery explained the risks and reactions to watch for again, and gave instructions to the nurse on duty. The nurses brought the dreaded pink bed/chair for one last outing, and I pushed the monstrosity around the fifth floor, staying on the floor in case the IVIG came from the pharmacy early. I helped Joe check his e-mail; he ate lunch and took a quick nap.

The neurology team came in and had to wake Joe to examine him. It was always interesting to watch them do their exams. They carried around several wooden sticks, the type that they use to swab your throat when testing for strep. They would take the stick out of the package, break it in half, and start poking the broken end into Joe's body. They would start near the top of the chest and work their way down to see where the feeling stopped. It looked very high tech. The nurse brought Tylenol and Benadryl, always given about an hour before the start of IVIG, to counteract bad reactions. When they tried to put the IV needle in, his veins rolled away and they had to stick him several times. They were finally able to get a vein in his left hand, a very bad place for a left-hander who was just becoming co-coordinated enough to feed himself. We were both disappointed and I knew that I would have to help him eat until the IV was taken out. They started the IVIG drip at 4:00, and I began my watch for adverse reactions. When Joe's dinner came, he was upset that I had to feed him again, but confident that he could put up with it for the next 28 hours.

Brian's wife came to see him around the time they were starting Joe's I.V. She had been feeling bad all day, had a high blood sugar reading at home, and soon left for the emergency room. She had been a diabetic for years and had a implanted insulin pump. We learned that the E.R. doctors suspected her insulin pump had stopped working. They decided to replace the pump's batteries and keep her overnight for observation. That seemed to be the last straw for Brian, he was sick with worry, with his entire family in the hospital. He convinced the doctor on duty to let him leave the floor long enough to go see his wife, but he the doctor wanted a nurse to go with him. All the nurses were busy, but since Joe was doing well, I volunteered to take him. The doctor agreed, if he wasn't gone long, so Brian got into a wheelchair, grabbed his IV pole, and we were off.

When we got to the emergency room, the nurses remembered Brian from when he had been admitted. We told them that I was his surrogate mom, borrowed from his Marine friend upstairs, and they let us go back to Jackie's room. Jackie was lying on a bed in one of the exam rooms. The doctor was in the room making notes on a clipboard and recognized Brian. Brian spoke to him briefly then went to Jackie's side. I gave him about 20 minutes, then dragged him away and started back to the elevators.

Brian and Jackie were a handsome couple and they obviously loved each other very much. "Someday you're going to laugh about this," I told him as I pushed his wheelchair down the hall. "How often do you have every member of your family in the same hospital at the same time? Not to mention, having some crazy lady pushing your wheelchair all over the hospital. Nobody will believe this story." That brought a weak chuckle from him, but I was certain that I was right. We checked in with the nurses and I helped Brian back into his bed. The trip had obviously worn him out.

I checked on Joe, who seemed to be doing well, then left for the Executive Dining Room. It was my third family dinner, and I was running late. When I got there, all the families were gone and the chefs were cleaning up. The room smelled of great food and I was starving. Even though the cooks were tired and ready to go home themselves, they seemed glad to see me as they handed me a take out box. I declined the meat entrée and filled my box with salad, roll, corn on the cob and chocolate cake. Thanking them once again for what I knew would be a wonderful meal, I hurried back and ate my dinner in Joe's room. The dinners were such a God-send for those of us who were in the hospital day in and day out, and they were always delicious.

Joe woke up hungry, so I warmed up some pasta from the refrigerator in the pantry and helped him eat. He wanted to send a letter to his fraternity in Springfield, so he dictated and I wrote it for him. He seemed to be tolerating the IVIG well. The first bottle of IVIG finished about 9:30 and the nurse started the second bottle. She gave Joe his night pills and he was ready to sleep. Brian was already asleep, so I gave Joe his IPOD, turned out the lights and left for the Navy Lodge. The air was crisp and cool, and a nice breeze was blowing. It had been quite a day.

Chapter 23

Saturday, October 21

Confrontation with Nurse

I got to the hospital early and found Joe sleeping. The IVIG seemed to be going well and his breakfast was sitting on his tray. I woke him up, warmed his breakfast in the microwave and helped him eat. While he was eating, Nurse Vedder came in, taking a few extra minutes to talk. She was one of our favorite nurses, always busy, and always there after the end of her shift. I asked her one day if she ever left on time, she thought for a minute and said "I can't remember the last time I left on time." I felt bad for all the nurses as they were understaffed on every shift. I wondered why the Navy didn't supply the hospital with more corpsmen and nurses, especially with all the injured coming back from the war. Everyone kept saying that the hospital had more patients than they'd had in years.

During the IVIG treatment, the nurses had to check Joe's vital signs every two hours, so he and Brian hadn't gotten much sleep the night before. After the normal doctor and therapists visits, I closed their door and went to the computer room. I returned when their lunches came, but they were still trying to sleep. I decided that lunch could wait, and put them both in the refrigerator. I tried to shoo all the nurses away so they could get some rest but it didn't last long, as the x-ray department called for Joe at noon. He had been having constipation, swelling and pressure in his abdomen, and the doctors had ordered an x-ray to see what was going on.

The nurse and I pushed Joe, in his bed, to the x-ray department on the 1st floor where we were surprised to hear that they wanted an x-ray with him sitting up. We explained to the x-ray technician that he wasn't able to sit up on his own but she said she had to get one x-ray with him sitting up. So, the three of us moved him from the bed to the x-ray table, pulled him into a sitting position, leaned his back against the back of the machine and propped pillows on both sides of him. It was a precarious position and I stayed next to him as the x-ray tech set everything up, then hurried behind the panel at the last second, ready to jump back out if he started to fall. Seconds later, the x-ray was done and we were able to lay him down for the next one. The tech checked to be sure the x-rays were good before we moved him back onto the bed for the trip back to his room. We were all worn out.

Brian was awake and they were both hungry, so I got their lunches out of the refrigerator, warmed them up, and they both ate well. They were immediately ready to go back to sleep, so I closed their door and went to Subway, getting my pizza to go. I ate in their room and was able to keep the nurses away for about 2 hours. They both slept well.

It was mid-afternoon when Dr. Pugh came in with the results of the x-rays, "The x-rays show a buildup of fecal material in the intestines but it's not impacted. We'll give potent laxatives and see if that clears it out."

"What?" Joe asked. He was still trying to wake up.

"You know, fecal material, crap actually. Nothing bad, we just have to clean it out."

"Oh," Joe mumbled, and went back to sleep. I smiled.

The nurse came in as Dr. Pugh was leaving, checked Joe's vitals and emptied the urine from the Foley bag. Joe went back to sleep, but not for long, as the nurse returned a few minutes later with a diaper and bottle of magnesium citrate drink. Joe drank it down, said it tasted like flat 7-up, and went back to sleep. He was even too tired to object to the diaper.

Joe and Brian both woke up when their dinner trays arrived, then the "poopy jokes" began! It was good to see that they still had their senses of humor. In short order, they were ready to sleep again, so I gave Joe his IPOD and shut their door as I left.

I ran into Michael's dad in the hospital lobby and stopped to talk to him for a few minutes. Michael was in ICU-18 when we first got to Bethesda and I'd talked to his dad a few times before. He told me that Michael had moved to 5 East, after spending 41 days in ICU. He was also in Iraq and was shot in the shoulder. The bullet did damage to his shoulder, and then hit his spine and lung. They had to remove half of his lung and use metal to put his spine back together. He had no feeling below the waist and the doctors didn't think the feeling would return; they were talking about sending him to the VA hospital in Tampa, which was near their home, for rehab. I was glad to hear that Michael had improved enough to get out of ICU and wished him well. The families I met at Bethesda were so strong!

As I walked to the Lodge, I got a call from the nursing home; Lou wanted to talk to me. It was good to receive only one call from him each day, allowing me to concentrate on helping Joe. I told him, again, where I was and what I was doing there. I told him that Joe

First One Home

was getting better. I don't think he remembered any of it. He told me that he would probably be gone on his business trip another 2 or 3 days. He said that the hotel wasn't the best but the lady behind the counter was nice. I asked if I could speak to her again and he handed the phone back to her, and then walked away. I thanked her for calling me. She said that Lou seemed fine during the day, confused in the afternoon and wandered the halls at night; not unusual for an Alzheimer's patient. He seemed content.

I ate my dinner in my room at the Lodge, and then walked back to the hospital. The sun was setting and it was a beautiful evening. I got back to Joe's room about 8:00 and was shocked to see that the IVIG had been stopped even though the bottle was not empty. Joe told me that Nurse C. had turned it off, saying the time was up, even though he told her it was supposed to run until it was gone. I was livid and went looking for her. Momma Bear was back. I found her at the nurse's station.

"I want to know why the IVIG infusion has been stopped in Room 4." I said.

"It was scheduled to run for 28 hours, so I stopped it when the 28 hours was up," she replied.

"No, it was scheduled to run until the bottle was empty and my son tried to tell you that before you stopped it. I want it restarted immediately."

"I can't do that without a doctor's approval."

"Then get a doctor up here."

"All the doctors have gone from this floor until tomorrow."

"Then you find another doctor, or better yet, you get Dr. Montgomery on the line. His number is on the orders. In fact, I want to talk to him myself."

"I can't do that," she glibly replied.

"Then I'll have you before the board on charges of medical malpractice and improper conduct and everyone at this nurse's station is a witness. I'm going to go get a paper and pen to write down everyone's name. You'll all be under subpoena on this one."

"No, wait. I'll find a doctor from another floor." I finally had her attention.

"Great, I'll be waiting in Room 4," I said, as I turned and walked away.

Within 15 minutes, Dr. Walton, the doctor on duty from 5 East came into Joe's room. I told him the situation and he left to check the orders. He was back within 5 minutes, had already ordered the IVIG to be restarted, and ordered it to run until the bottle was empty. I thanked him for his help and he went back to his unit.

Joe smiled and said, "You know, mom, you can be a bitch sometimes."

Brian said "You go, Barb, someone needs to stand up to these people."

I was thrilled to get both compliments!

Joe told me that, when Nurse C. had stopped the IVIG and flushed the IV with saline, she pushed the plunger very fast and it hurt. His hand still hurt. I knew that could be bad, but I hoped for the best. Soon, the corpsman came in to hook the IVIG back up but it started burning as soon as she started it. Just what I was afraid of, the vein had been blown. They would have to put in another IV. The corpsman tried twice but was unable to get another IV started. Finally, at 9:45, they called for Dr. Walton again and he was able to get the IV in and the IVIG was restarted.

Nurse C. was one of the regular night nurses, a Navy nurse from Puerto Rico who had done a couple of other marginal things. Now, she was Number One on my radar screen and I vowed to watch her every move. Brian thought we should ask that she no longer be allowed in their room but with the shortage of nurses, I was afraid to do that. Sometimes it would take 20 minutes for a nurse to appear after the call button was pushed and I was afraid of even longer waits. We decided not to do anything yet.

This incident was just one of many that I observed, one more reason it was so very important for all the patients to have someone with them to advocate for them. They were all much to sick to handle these types of situations on their own.

Even with all the commotion, and no luck in the bowel movement department, there was good news. Joe reported that he could feel the sensation when urinating. Nurse C. came in at 11:30 gave him a suppository and he said he could feel that too. That was GREAT news. Brian was also taking magnesium citrate, and the "poopy jokes" were rampant. It was good to hear them laugh, and so the contest was on — who would have the first successful "poop"?

By midnight, they were sleepy again so I gave Joe his IPOD, turned out the lights, shut their door, and left for the Navy Lodge. There was coolness in the air and I could smell the sweet smells of autumn. The darkness enveloped me as I moved up the hill.

Chapter 24

Sunday, October 22

Visitors and Phone Calls

The day began with my normal walk down the hill toward the hospital, I thought about all that had happened over the past 3 weeks. At home, my neighbors had not only picked up the mail and given it to my folks when they came to town, they'd also kept the lawn mowed and watched for unusual happenings. My folks had driven the 85 miles into town several times to pick up my mail, keep my bills paid, water the plants, adjust the air conditioner, and clean out the refrigerator. They'd visited Lou at the nursing home and tried to keep him calm. My good friends, Julie and Doris, had visited him too.

At school, Angie, my substitute, had done what she could and other employees had helped her with the jobs she wasn't trained to do. I was sure it had been a real learning experience for her. Everyone was helping out and I was getting e-mails with words of encouragement every day. A few people would call me, but most sent e-mails and I sent a mass e-mail each day to keep everyone informed. My sisters in Tulsa had stepped up to the plate, done all they could to help Lou, then drove him back to Springfield when he needed more care than they could give. Now their lives were getting back to normal.

The trees were starting to turn those lovely yellow, red and orange colors of fall and I stopped to take a couple of pictures as I walked. I wondered how much longer we'd be at Bethesda.

When I arrived at the hospital, Joe's door was closed and a "DND" sign was taped to it. There was something new. I went in quietly to find Joe sleeping, the IVIG bottle finished and hanging in the corner. The IV was still in his hand, but had no tubing attached. Brian whispered to me that they were both exhausted from being awaked so many times during the night. When the nurse had come in at 6 am to take Joe's blood sample (which they did every morning), he told her to go away and hid his arms under the covers. There had been a rebellion in Room 4 — thus explaining the "Do Not Disturb" sign on the door. I smiled; baby bear and friend were rising up!

Nurse Waddill quietly came into the room; she was a wonderful nurse and one of our favorites. She was actually a corpsman, and just 19 years old, but very knowledgeable with great people skills. She had been in the Navy for over a year and it was easy to see that she loved her work. Glancing at Brian, she told me that there was still no success in the BM department for either patient and the plan was to give them both enemas if nothing happened that day. She brought some warm packs, plastic bags that warm up when you twist them, and we put them on Joe's stomach.

Dr. Miller had already been there and was encouraged that Joe had feeling down to his naval! Dr. Fung came in, was concerned about Joe's morning revolt, and said that he might be depressed. Well, that would make sense, he was lying in bed, unable to roll over by himself, the nurses wouldn't listen to him, and he couldn't poop, I would be depressed too. Dr. Fung was a genius.

When the doctors left, Joe was hungry and grumpy. I warmed up his breakfast, and helped him eat it. He was upset about having to give blood so often and being stuck with needles in general. I reminded him that they had to get his vital signs every two hours while he was on the IVIG and, although he understood, he still didn't like it. As soon as he finished eating, he was ready to go back to sleep, so I gave him his IPOD and stayed with him to try to keep the nurses away.

They took Brian out for an ultrasound on his leg, which would tell them which parts of his burn needed skin grafts. He was scheduled for skin grafts the following day. I had seen the burn up close, and it was a nasty one. The highest point was mid-hip, the lowest point at the top of the knee, and about 10 inches wide at the widest point. He was obviously in a lot of pain and gladly took the pain killers the nurses offered.

While Brian was gone, the nurses came in to give Joe an enema and I went out in the hall while they worked with him.

While I was standing in the hall, MGen. Jones, with the Semper Fi Fund, walked by and introduced himself. I had heard of the fund from the other parents and was glad to meet him. He gave me a form, and encouraged me to fill it out and turn it in. He was a bit upset that we had been there three weeks and he hadn't met us yet. He apologized repeatedly for not knowing that we were there. I had noticed that most visitors went to 5 East, the surgical ward, and few ever made it to 5 Center, the medical ward, and overflow ward for 5 East. Because of that, the wounded who were on 5 Center missed out on many things and it was just luck that had brought him down the hall at the exact moment I was standing outside Joe's room.

During the rest of our time at Bethesda I would mention this to several people who brought visitors to see the young men on 5

Center. One group that I was not able to contact was the USO. They brought entertainers to 5 East every Thursday, but none of them ever came to 5 Center. It was a shame that the young Marines who happened to get a room on 5 Center never got to meet the singers and actors. These celebrities seemed to boost the morale of the patients so much.

When the Red Team came, we talked about the DND sign on Joe's door. They told us that they would ask the nurses to do everything they needed to do in one trip (vitals, medications, blood draws, sponge bath, etc.) which would allow both patients to get more rest. They were also ordering more laxatives for each of them.

Brian came back from his ultrasound and was in a lot of pain. He said it was brutal because they had to roll the ultrasound wand over all parts of his burn — even the parts that were third degree! But after lunch, the "poopy jokes" started again and I escaped to get lunch myself.

When I returned, Sgt. Major Truillo and Commander Landro were there talking to Joe. They were with the 25th Marines, the unit Joe's group had replaced in Iraq and I learned that Joe had actually ridden in Commander Landro's humvee while he was in Iraq. They had a nice visit and it was interesting to listen to them. Joe was excited to have visitors, someone he knew, and stayed awake talking excitedly after they left, while I ate my lunch.

I had just finished eating when Brian had success in the bathroom with his "poopy" problem! It stunk up the whole room and the "poppy jokes" began again. Joe said, "I'm happy for you man, but since I'm stuck over here by the window with no way to get out of the room — and away from your success story — it kind of sucks too."

We all had a good laugh, and the nurse brought in some air freshener — bless her.

Joe got another bottle of magnesium citrate as soon as he got it down, he promptly fell asleep. While he was sleeping I got a phone call from my parents who were at the nursing home visiting Lou. My friend, Julie, was there when they arrived and Lou had told her that he was in the hospital because he'd had a heart attack. He also told her that Joe & I were on our way to see him and she should wait for us. I talked to Lou for a minute and his story to me was that he was still on a business trip but would be ready to come home soon. Later, I would learn that my friend, Doris, had also gone to see him that day — so he had a busy day.

While I was on the phone, Brian decided to take a walk down the hall. He ran into a friend in the hall and this friend was visiting a patient in a nearby room who had been wounded in Iraq. Brian went into that patient's room with his friend — and was discovered there by one of the nurses. It became a <u>major</u> issue as his burn was uncovered and burns are easily infected. To complicate matters, the patient he went to see was infected with acinebactor, a nasty Iraqi bacteria that many of the guys came home with. Acinebactor was the main reason that all visitors had to wear gowns & gloves until the patient tested negative. The problem with acinebactor is that it is resistant to most antibiotics, so infections are hard to treat, and it can be lethal. The nurses were VERY upset with Brian and sent him directly to the shower. They bagged up the clothes he was wearing in one of those red bags marked "biohazard", and when Jackie came in to see him, gave it to her with special washing instructions.

It was mid afternoon when the nurse brought in the dreaded pink chair. It was a real pain to use, but the only way to get many of the patients up and moving around. It was cumbersome and cost several thousand dollars but the nurses liked it because it lessened the strain on their backs. I tolerated it because it was the only way to get Joe out and about. We didn't go far, just to the computer room to check our e-mails. Joe was getting more control over his fingers and was able to slowly type on his own. He enjoyed his independence and I enjoyed watching.

We went back to Joe's room when we saw the dinner cart go by, and he ate while sitting in the pink chair. Shortly after getting back into bed, the much anticipated B.M. came. You would think that he'd discovered a cure for cancer. Everyone was so glad to see his bowels moving again. The nurses didn't even complain when they changed the diaper. He and Brian had fun with the "poopy jokes" once again.

Nurse Vedder came in with Joe's insulin shot, giving it in his belly where he couldn't feel the needle stick. I messaged his feet and calves with lotion and noticed that his leg would jump if I put the lotion on his feet without warming it up in my hands first. I also noticed that his leg would jerk when I messaged certain spots on his feet. I hoped that it was a good sign. Andy called and talked to Joe while I was doing the message. It was nice to get calls from his buddies back home.

Nurse C. came in at 7:30 and took his vitals. She wanted to clean the IV but Joe wouldn't let her touch it (smart boy). I told her to take it out as Joe wouldn't be getting any more transfusions, and she left to check the doctor's orders. I was a little concerned about her being the night nurse, but knew that she would be doing one visit around bedtime and wouldn't return until 6 am, and both Joe & Brian seemed to be able to handle her.

Brian was scheduled for skin grafts the next morning and was very nervous. When he first came in, he was pumped full of morphine, then they switched to dilaudid. He seemed to need more and more dilaudid, so they tried to change back to morphine but it didn't seem to work as well and they switched him back to dilaudid. Over the past few days, he had become more and more agitated. I'm not a doctor, but it seemed to me that he was building up immunity.

After Nurse C's bedtime visit, I put the pumpers on Joe's legs, gave him his IPOD, turned out the lights and closed the door. Brian was ready to go to sleep too. It was a cold night and I was glad to have my fleece jacket as I walked up the hill toward the Navy Lodge.

When I got to the Lodge, there was a family checking in, 3 adults and 3 kids. We went down in the elevator together, and I learned that they were in a room near mine. I also learned that the group was a married couple, their daughter, the wife's sister, and her two kids. The kids were extremely polite and well mannered and they told me that they were there because the couple's son had been wounded in Iraq.

Their son was in 1/24 Marines, Charlie Company and his humvee had been hit by an IED; of the four men in the vehicle, two were wounded and two were killed. Both the wounded had been sent to Bethesda and the other man had lost both his legs. Their son had injuries to both legs, one of which was held together with lots of metal.

Joe was also in the 1/24 Marines but he served in Headquarters Company, so he didn't know many of the Charlie Company guys; and he didn't know any of these guys. The 1/24 Marines that went to Iraq was made up of several units, most of them were from Michigan but they also had guys from Missouri, Ohio and Arkansas. One of the big problems with a group like that was getting them to gel together and work as a team, after such a short training period together. This was another nice family torn apart by war.

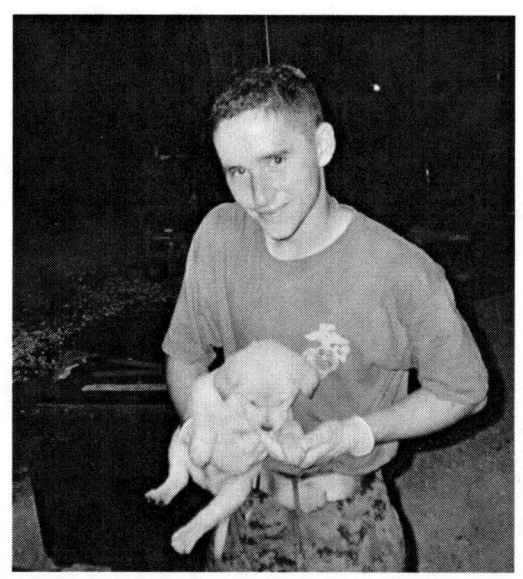

While Joe's unit was in New Orleans in 2005, he helped out at an animal rescue shelter.

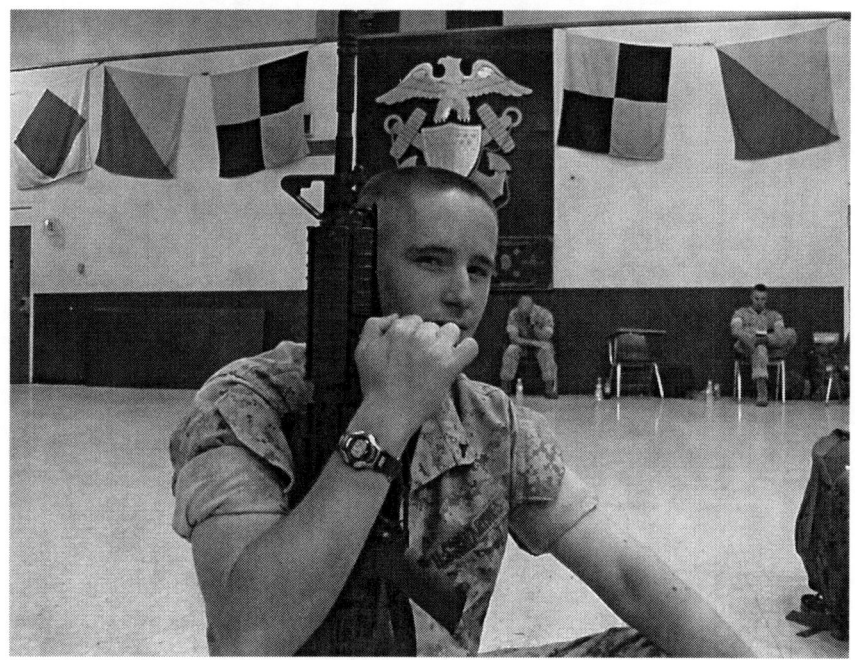

Joe between flights on his way to Iraq in September 2006.

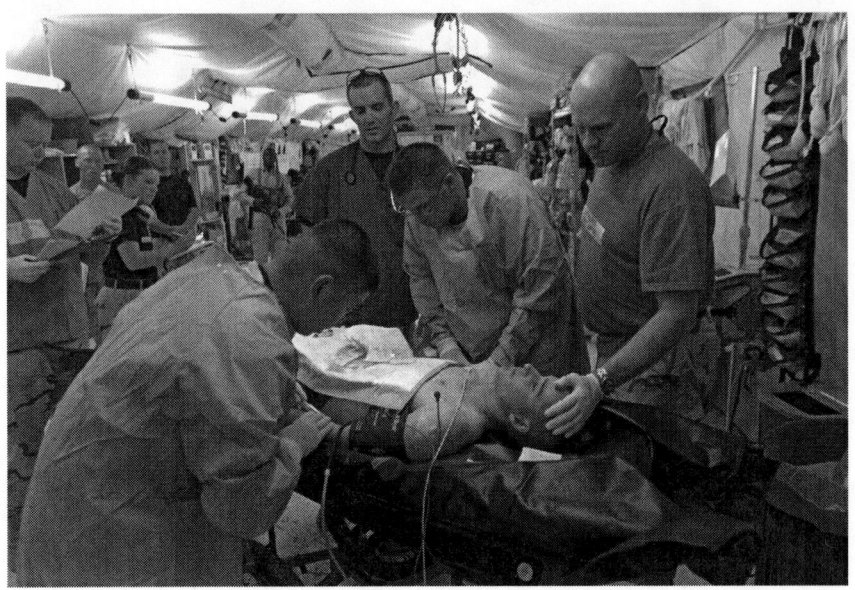

Just nine days after arriving in Iraq, Joe was brought to this emergency room in Balad. The chaplain places his hand on Joe's head as the doctor and medics attempt to make a diagnosis.

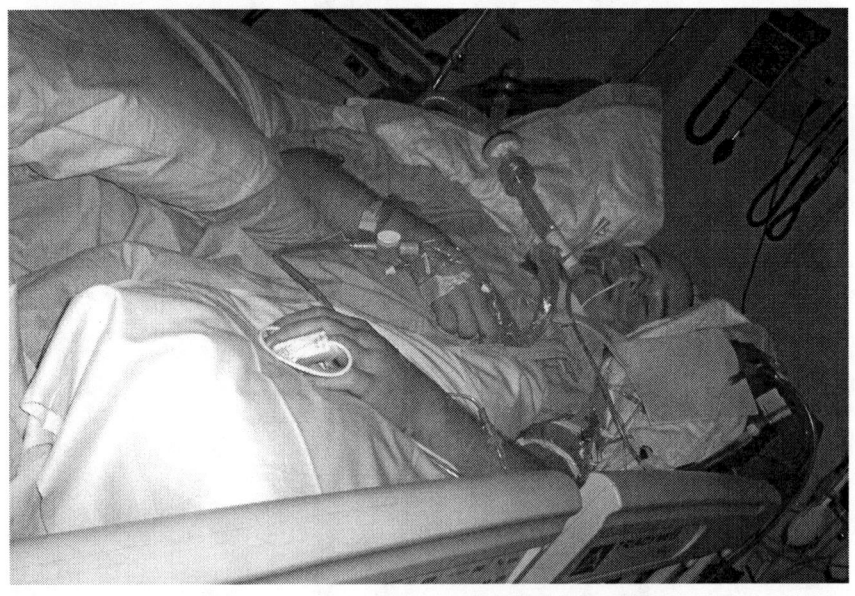

When I first saw Joe in Landstuhl, Germany, he was in a coma and on life support.

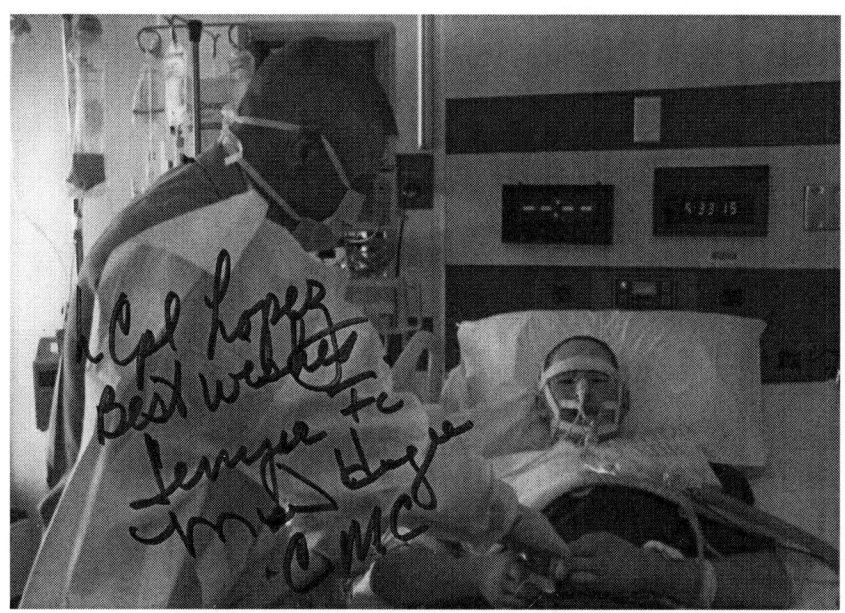

Just days after arriving at Bethesda Naval Medical Center, U. S. Marine Corps Commandant Hagee visited Joe in his ICU room and gave him one of his coins.

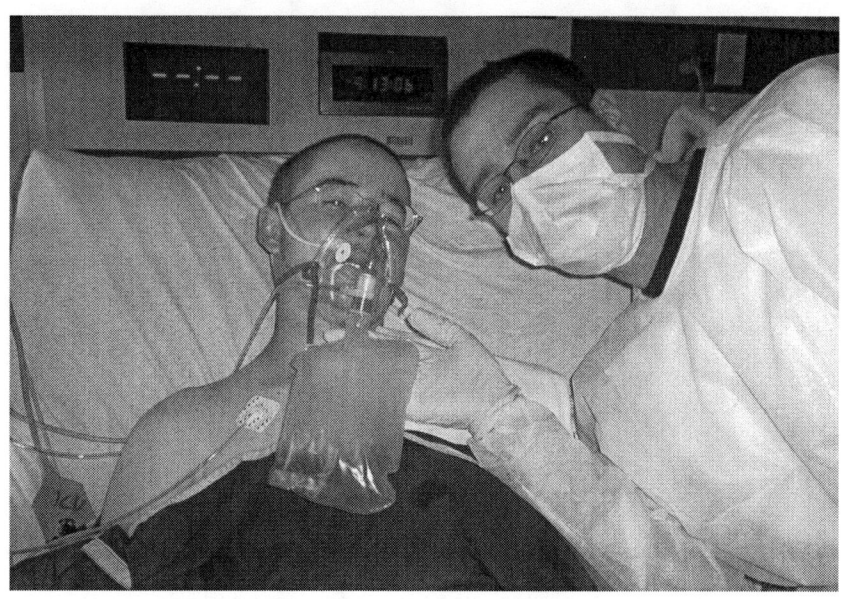

Still in ICU, as Joe began to improve, he posed for a picture with his brother, Steven.

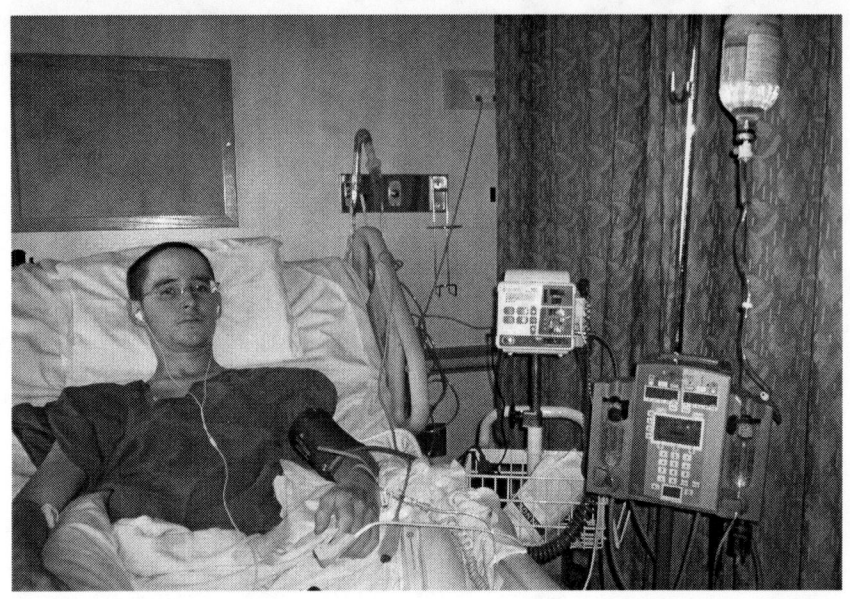

After moving out of ICU, Joe had a second IVIG infusion, and eventually had a total of 4 treatments.

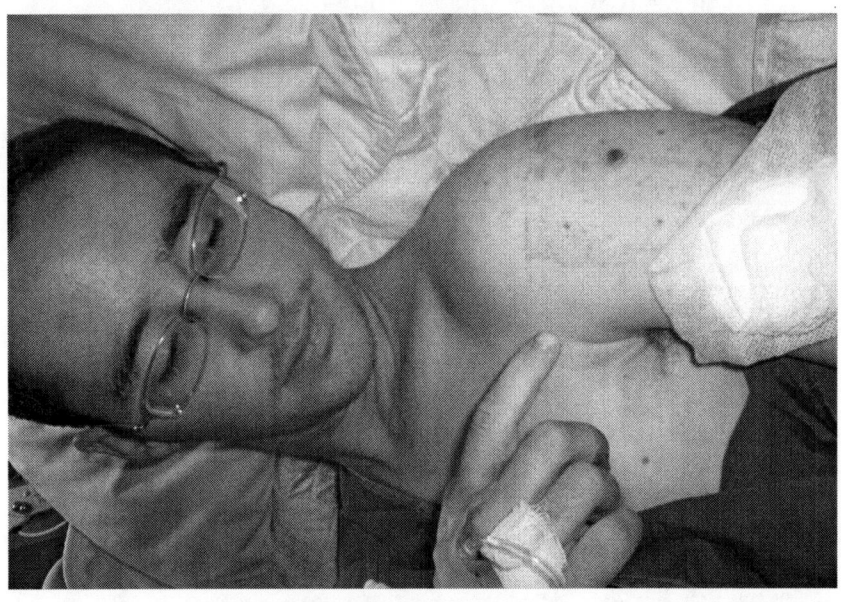

The hospital staff cleaned and re-covered Joe's smallpox site each day until the scab fell off.

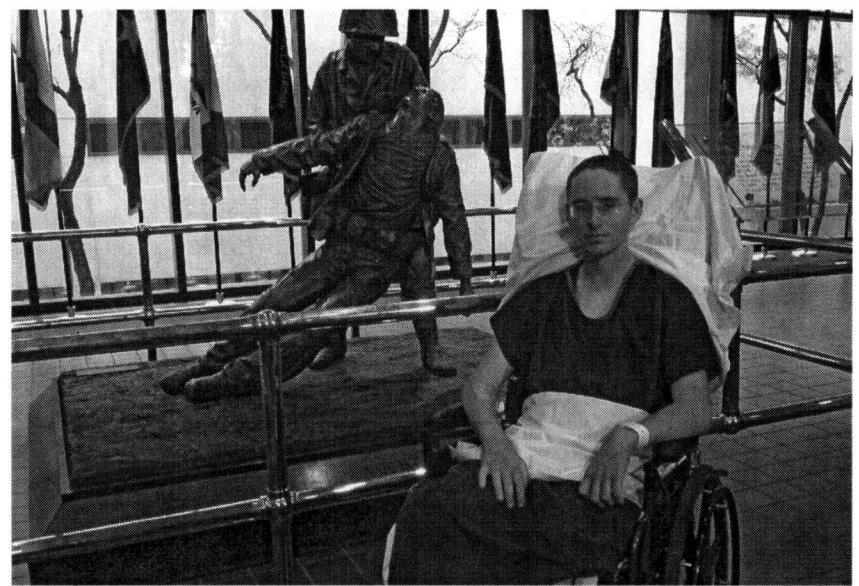

For Joe's first trip off the floor, I took him to the lobby to show him this statue of a Navy medic pulling an injured Marine to safety. Every day, as I came and went from the hospital, I was encouraged by this statue.

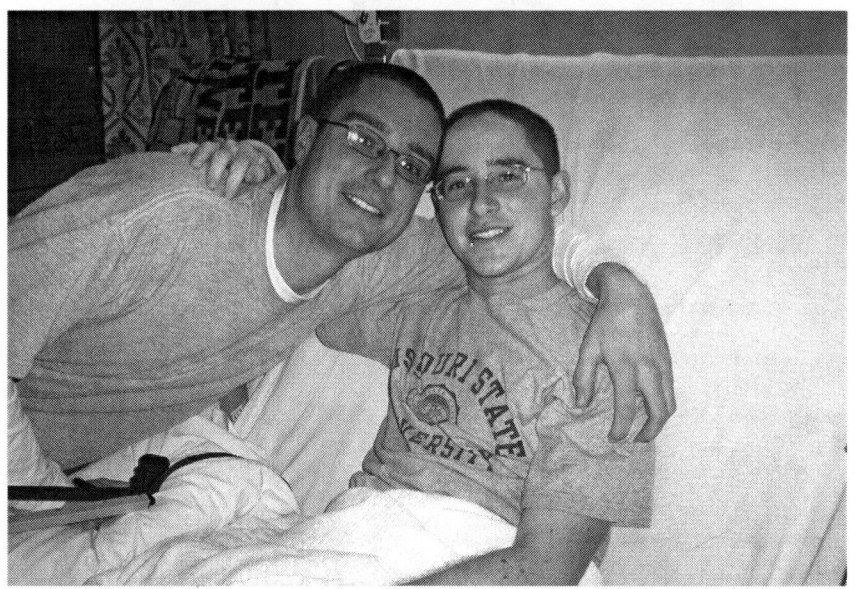

Steven and Joe on his second trip to Bethesda. Steven was so happy to see his brother free of all tubes and I.V.'s.

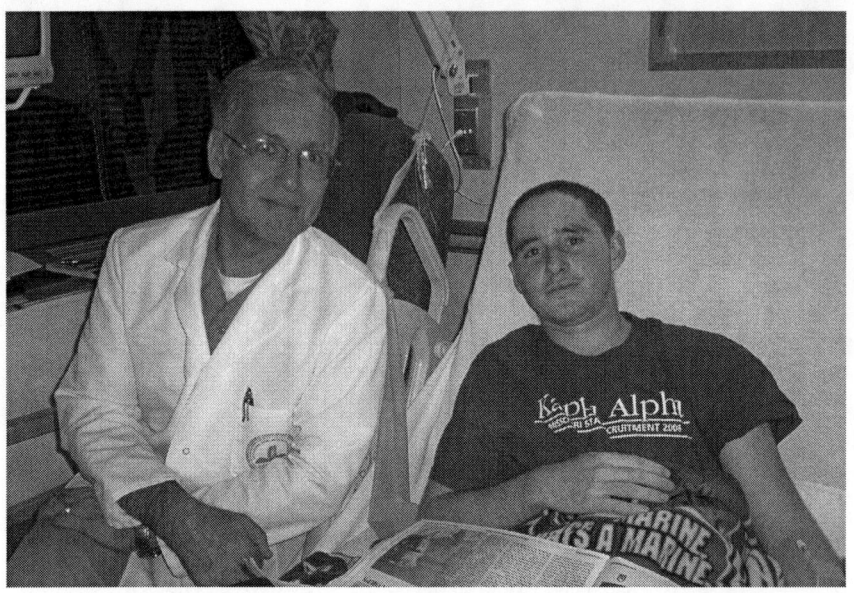

Dr. Montgomery, who saved Joe's life, posed with Joe for this picture the day before we left Bethesda.

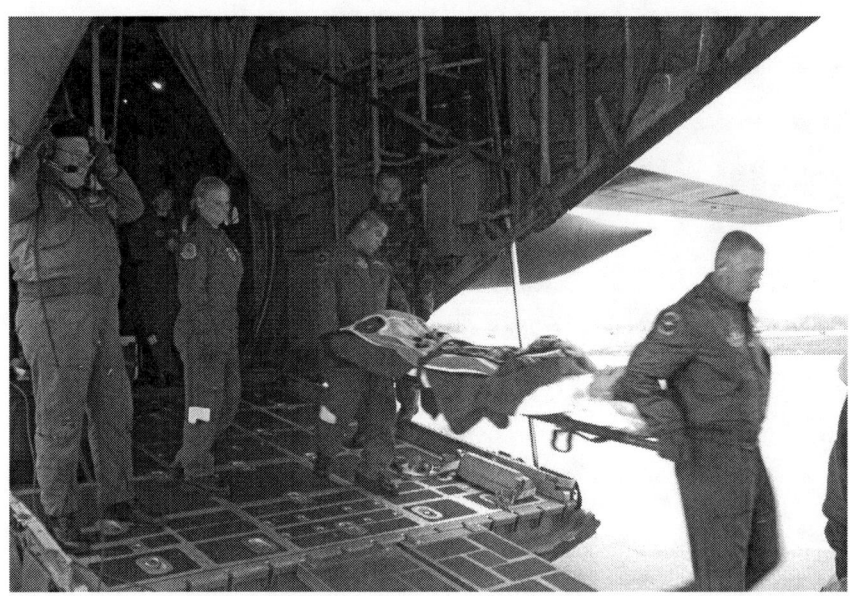

When our plane arrived in Springfield, the Air Force personnel carried Joe to the waiting St. John's Hospital Ambulance.

First One Home

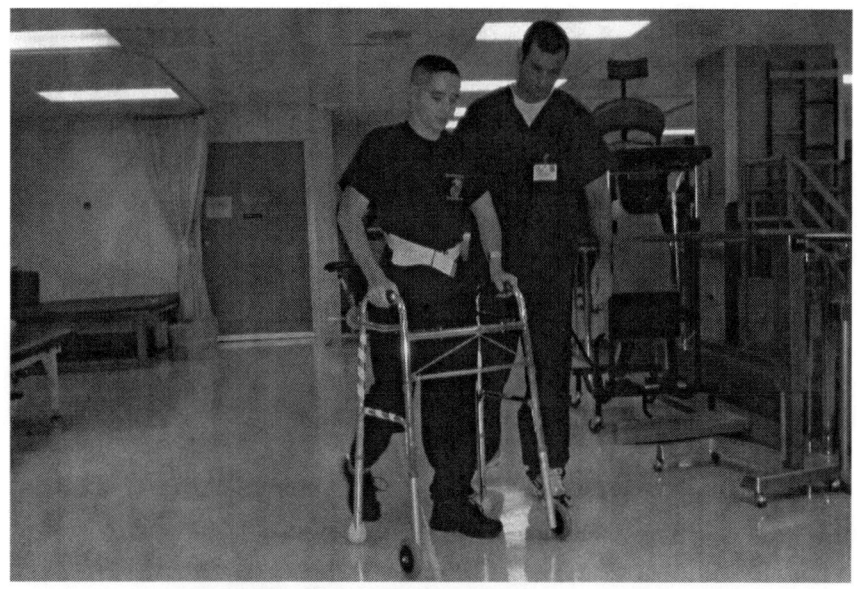

Joe worked hard in physical therapy for over year, as both in-patient and out-patient, to learn to walk again.

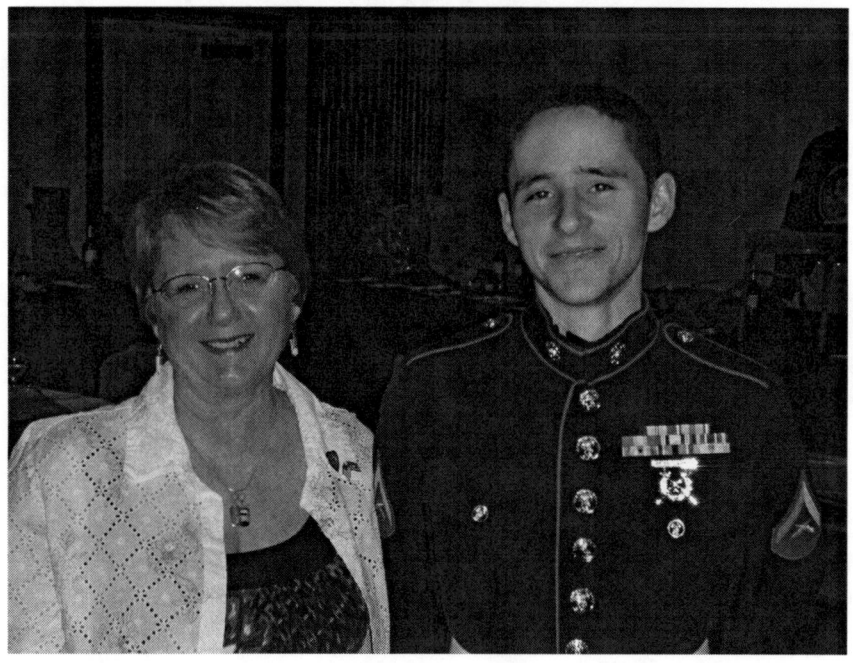

Barbara and Joe at the Marine Parents conference in 2008.

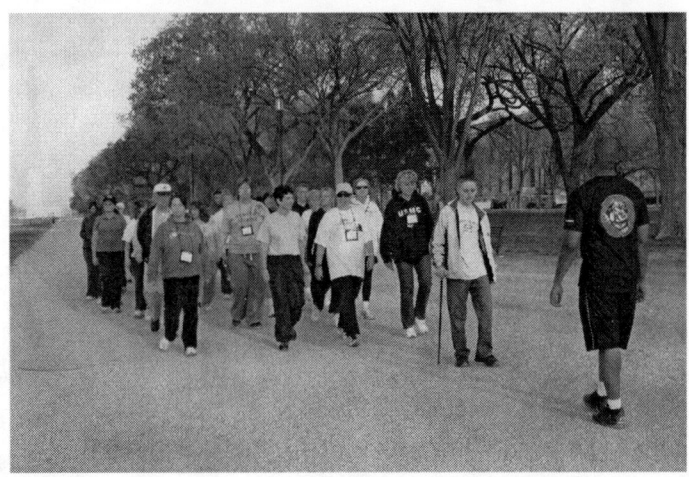

Joe, walking with a cane, leading the group of Marine parents on a walk at the Marine Parents conference in 2008.

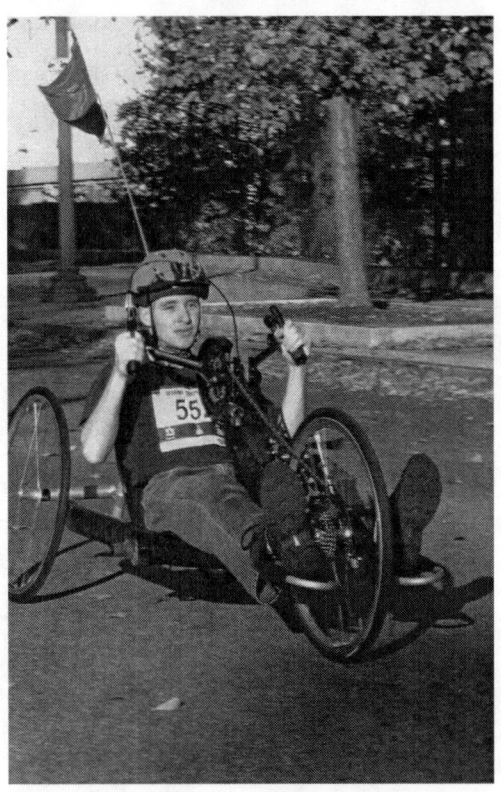

Joe riding his hand cycle in the Marine Corps Marathon. Addition pictures can be viewed at firstonehome.com

Chapter 25

Monday, October 23

Haircut

The day began on a good note. The night of uninterrupted sleep seemed to help as Joe was in good spirits. His vital signs were good, the physical therapist worked on his arms and legs and even sat him up on the edge of the bed for the first time. His abdominal muscles were getting stronger every day. Dr Montgomery and the neurologist were pleased to see that Joe was able to move his legs and toes and had more feeling overall. He seemed to have feeling above the naval and below the knees, but still numbness in the middle section of his body.

I ran into Lt. Marino, the head of nursing, in the hall and he asked how things were going. He was very professional and genuinely concerned about his patients. I told him that I had asked for Joe's IV to be taken out the day before, the doctors had approved it, but nothing had been done. He checked on it right away then went right to Joe's room and took it out himself. Joe was certainly glad to get that over with.

I put lotion on Joe's feet and calves and was pleased to see that he was able to move both legs and big toes and also felt the coldness of the lotion. Then the doctors and therapists began their daily visits.

I stayed with Joe while he ate his lunch, and then went to the galley for my own lunch. I saw the Lang family, from last night, and they told me they had seen their son in ICU and thought he was doing well. The other injured Marine was also doing well.

Later, I would learn the names of the two men who had been killed in the attack, and was relieved that Joe didn't know either of them. I knew he felt guilty that he wasn't there fighting along side his brothers and each time a member of the 1/24 Marines came into the hospital, I was afraid it would be one of his good friends. Somehow, it didn't seem so bad if it was a stranger.

After lunch, Joe had physical therapy, then the nurses helped him into the dreaded pink chair, gave him his meds and insulin shot, and cleared him to leave the floor for a couple of hours. Soon we were on our way to the elevators, with me pushing and pulling, huffing and puffing, trying to keep the chair going in a semi-straight line.

Joe had been asking for a haircut for some time, and I knew that the Barber Shop was in the basement, directly across from Subway. There were 2 ramps between the elevator and the barber shop, nice long ramps if one is pushing a regular wheelchair — but a real obstacle course if one is pushing the dreaded pink chair. I was a bit worried about Joe, with his weak abdominal muscles, afraid he could tip forward and fall out of the chair when we started going downhill — and I wasn't at all sure that I could push him back UP the hill in the heavy chair once we made it down — but there was no elevator. When we got to the first ramp, he said he would be fine and promised to tell me if he started to fall forward, so I took a deep breath and started down the ramp.

Suddenly, my worst fears were realized as Joe fell forward and said "Help me, I'm falling, I'm falling!"

I tried to stop the chair, while stepping to the side and grabbing one shoulder to keep him upright. Of course, the chair was heavy, it rolled downhill on its own and I was totally helpless against it. My only hope was to keep him upright until we came to a stop at the bottom and I tried with all my strength to hold him up.

Just before we got to the bottom of the incline, he pulled himself upright, looked over at me, grinned, and said "Gotcha!"

"You little shit, were you playing with me all along? Do you realize I almost killed myself trying to stop this stupid chair and keep your happy butt from falling on the ground? I ought a kick your butt right here in front of all these people walking by!" He just laughed and laughed, until I started laughing too. What a brat!

We made it safely to the barber shop where the barber moved one of the barber chairs off to the side and we pushed Joe and the dreaded pink chair into position. Now the pink chair is basically a bed that sits up, so there is a part of the chair that is directly behind the head. It was a real challenge for the barber to get to the hair on the back of Joe's head. He had to maneuver the clippers just so, and Joe had to lean his head forward as far as he could. As the hair fell away, I noticed that there was a round spot on the back of Joe's head with absolutely no hair growing inside it, about the size of a silver dollar. The barber worked his magic, even within the confines of the pink chair, and when he was done, Joe had a high and tight Marine haircut. He looked good, even with the little hairless circle in the back, and it boosted his spirits to look like a Marine again.

We stopped in at the computer room where Joe checked his e-mails and answered them himself; he was getting more and more control over his fingers and it was good to see him using the computer by himself again. It was one of his favorite things.

When we got back to Joe's room, we found that they had taken his fancy ICU bed away and replaced it with a regular hospital bed. He didn't seem to mind, and settled in for a quiet evening of reading and watching TV.

Jackie came in to see Brian, and when she left, she brought the chair she'd been using to Joe's side of the room. She knew that I spent most of the day there and wanted me to have it; and she was afraid that someone might take it to another room if she left it on Brian's side of the room. The chair said ICU on it, but was nothing like the metal, folding chairs that had been in Joe's ICU room. It was on wheels, reclined and had a foot rest. I gladly took it, knowing that I would be able to recline and nap with it. Jackie was feeling much better and had been to see their baby, who was also doing well

Dr. Montgomery came by at 8:30 (he worked late quite often) and told us that he would like to bring two doctors from the Vaccine Health Center to meet Joe. He had been consulting with them about Joe's case since the first day, and explained that the VHC was started to track vaccination problems, to help make vaccinations safer, and their office was at Walter Reed. Joe wiggled one of his big toes and Dr. Montgomery was pleased to see it. He also talked about a third, and maybe even fourth dose of IVIG.

At 9:45, the night nurse came for her last visit. She took Joe's vitals, gave meds, checked blood sugar & diaper and gave him an insulin shot. Then she went to Brian and took care of everything he needed. Before their rebellion, she would have come into the room at least 6 times to accomplish the same thing. I was proud of their rebellious attitudes. I helped Joe brush his teeth, gave him his IPOD, turned out the lights, and closed the door. With any luck, they'd be able to sleep, undisturbed until 6 am.

It was almost time to extend my military orders, so I stopped by the Marine Liaison office and made arrangements to do the paperwork, then went back to the Navy Lodge and washed clothes again. I was very sleepy by the time it was finished.

Chapter 26

Tuesday, October 24

Shave

I went directly to the Marine Liaison office where Sgt. Barillo helped me with the paperwork to extend my orders until December 1, but I hoped I wouldn't be staying that long.

When I got to Joe's room, I learned that his steroids had been lowered to 65 mg, and the doctors had begun their visits. Joe's urine had protein in it and Dr. Fung said they would be watching it, and might even send him for an ultrasound of his kidneys. He was concerned that it could be a sign of kidney damage, which is one of the side effects of IVIG. His feet and legs were twitching more than the day before and, in the next bed, Brian is impatiently waiting for surgery.

Brian was pretty agitated by the time lunch came. He wasn't allowed to eat before surgery so he hadn't had breakfast and didn't get lunch. He was hungry, wanted to get the surgery over with and couldn't imagine why they hadn't come for him yet. Joe felt guilty to be eating and asked me to pull the curtain between them.

First One Home

When Joe finished eating, I went to eat my lunch and ran into Mr. Johnson — the guy we had met in Germany. His son had been on 5 East for some time and was ready to go to rehab. They would be leaving the next morning for the VA Hospital in Richmond, Virginia. The family lived in Texas and they hoped to be transferred to a hospital there after a short time in Richmond. I wished him the best and hurried to the galley before their closing time.

When I got back to Joe's room, he was asleep. Brian was still there and he was even more agitated. He was talking about walking out of the hospital, and going home, as he striped the sheets off the bed, piling them in the corner. He called Jackie, told her to come and get him, and started putting on his socks. About that time Nurse Flannigan walked in and she was livid! She had just changed the sheets that morning while he was in the shower and ordered him to put them back on the bed and get in it as they were on the way to get him for surgery. He calmed down and apologized to her for messing up his bed. She left the room in a huff and he started putting things back in order. It was like watching a mother scold her child for misbehaving. I knew it was hard for him to stand on his injured leg but he managed to get the sheets back on the bed and crawled into it.

While Brian was working on his bed, Dr. Barsozek, Dr. Fu and two interns came in to examine Joe. They talked about the possibility of doing another IVIG treatment or plasma pheresis. I already knew that plasma pheresis was the "usual" treatment for ADEM. The IVIG treatment that Dr. Montgomery had been using was new, and many neurologists felt that it was "experimental". Many of the neurologists wanted to go back to the "usual treatment" even though Joe was making great progress with IVIG. The doctors also talked about sending Joe to the Tampa VA Hospital for rehab but I asked them to check on a hospital in Springfield or at least one in the state of Missouri.

There were three Marines from Joe's unit at Bethesda but Joe hadn't known any of them while they were in Iraq. We heard that one of the Marines from his unit in Kansas City (Kelly) had been shot a week earlier, but would stay in Iraq while he healed, so we decided that it couldn't have been very bad. He was the first of Joe's friends to be wounded. Kelly had been shot in the buttocks by a drive-by shooter (bet he never lives that down, Joe was already making jokes). We would learn later that the bullet had actually grazed his spine, so it was more serious than we'd thought.

At 2:00, the corpsmen mercifully arrived to take Brian to surgery.

During the quiet while Brian was gone, the nurses came in to bathe and change Joe, then a corpsman came in with a razor and shaving cream. Since he was on blood thinners and his hands were shaky, they hadn't let him shave by himself before. The corpsman stayed in the room just in case he cut himself but he did just fine, enjoying another slice of independence.

Not long after he finished shaving, a new physical therapist came in and helped Joe into the recliner chair that Jackie had given me. He told us that the chair was meant for Joe anyway. Apparently, whoever brought had left it on the wrong side of the room! We reclined it back as far as it would go and I pushed Joe over to the computer room, it was wonderfully easy to push but I had to be careful to keep it reclined. Since his abdominal muscles were still weak, I was afraid he could topple out if he was sitting straight up, so I was very careful as I pushed it. When we got to the computer room, I was able to push the chair right up to the computer table, and then set the back of the chair up straight. It was a lot easier than the pink chair and Joe seemed to like it better too.

While we were at the computers, a group came in and started to set up tables for a buffet dinner. The dinner was provided for the families by the Armed Forces Foundation, and we enjoyed the food and conversation, staying for a long time.

Brian was back from surgery when we returned to Joe's room. They hadn't done the skin graft as the burn area was too irritated, so they would try again on Friday. Brian's mother was a nurse, and because of that, he had enough medical knowledge that they had allowed him to clean his wound himself. Apparently, he had been cleaning it too often, they put him on a cleaning schedule so he'd be ready on Friday.

The nurse came in to clean and change Joe's catheter, so I went to the computer room to check my e-mails. There was one other person at the computers and, after a few minutes, she turned and asked me if I was from Missouri.

"Yes, I'm from Springfield", I answered.

"Well, I'm from Columbia", she said.

"Are you Connie?"

"Yes, I heard that there was someone else from Missouri here, but I hadn't gotten a chance to meet you", she said.

I told her that I had read the article about her son on our return flight from Germany but hadn't had a chance to look for her either. We had both been too busy taking care of our boys. Connie told me that her son, John, was doing better and they would be leaving in the morning. He had actually been wounded three times and had received 3 purple hearts. The first time, it was a piece of shrapnel in his wrist. They cut it out and he returned to duty the next day. The second time, a bullet went into the front of his arm, near the shoulder, and then exited the back of his arm. It didn't hit anything vital and he was back on duty in a couple of days. By then, everyone was calling him "Lucky" and "Bullet Magnet", but the third wound was much worse. A sniper's bullet went into his head, just below his helmet, causing damage to his eye, ear, nerves and brain. They had done surgery on his brain and had implanted a piece of gold into his eyelid to weigh it down so it would close. The nerve damage caused one side of his face to droop, much like someone who had had a stroke, and the doctors were sending him to the VA hospital in Tampa for rehab. I gave Connie my e-mail address and she promised to keep in touch. As the weeks progressed, we would become e-mail buddies.

Just as I was leaving, Debbie came into the room and Connie introduced us. The two ladies had become good friends while their sons were healing. Debbie was from Michigan and her son, David, had leg and hand wounds. I would get to know them well over the next few weeks.

Joe & Brian were both watching TV when I got back to their room. I gave Joe his nightly foot and leg rub and their nurse came in to take vitals and give night meds. They were both sleepy, so I gave Joe his IPOD, turned out the lights, shut the door, and left for the Lodge. It was a nice walk and another cool night, a nice ending to Joe's first week out of ICU.

CHAPTER 27

Wednesday, October 25

Lots of Visitors

As I entered the hospital, I noticed another film crew in the lobby. There were often film crews there and, after awhile, I barely noticed them. I would learn later that this particular crew was filming for Bob Woodruff's television special.

It was a normal, busy morning in Joe's room, including a sponge bath given by a student nurse, then the parade of visitors began. Corpsman Walling was working on the other side of the hall but she stopped in to say hello. Joe moved his right leg for her.

Corporal Lopes, one of the Marine Liaisons, came by with General Wilson, a 2 star general. He was very nice, talked to Joe about his illness and wished him well. It was good for Joe to talk to people like the General; they raised his spirits and gave him hope.

When Joe was in ICU, he had a hallucination about Corporal Lopes, imagining that he was trying to kill him. One day, when Lopes came into his room, Joe asked him why he had tried to kill him and Lopes was really taken aback! They had a nice talk and, from then on, when Lopes would come around, Joe would say to him: "You're the one who tried to kill me when I was in ICU". They would always laugh, and I think they might have become good friends if they'd met under different circumstances.

Next came the physical therapist, who helped Joe into the reclining chair at the end of his treatment. When the nurse checked Joe's blood sugar, she said he didn't need any insulin. He was thrilled to hear that, as he was starting to feel the needles in his stomach – it was a good sign.

After lunch the Chaplain of the Marine Corps and the highest enlisted Chaplain came in. We had a nice visit with them, they each gave Joe a coin, and they were most encouraging.

After dinner, Colonel Dunahoe of the 1/24 Marines came by. He told us that there were 4 Marines from the 1/24 at Bethesda and more were on the way. He seemed frustrated as he told us, "It's been a tough week". He told Joe that his next mission would be to South America and he was looking for Spanish-speaking Marines to go with him. He was hopeful that Joe might be well enough to go with them, but seemed a little disappointed to hear that he didn't speak Spanish. It was encouraging to Joe to think that the Marines still wanted him.

After the Colonel left, I gave Joe a backrub. His muscles were tight and he had feeling in his back at a lower level than last week, even below the T6 area, which was where the neurology team said his feeling currently stopped.

By 9:15, Brian was asleep and Joe was also ready to sleep. I gave him his IPOD, turned out the lights, and walked to the Navy Lodge. The days were so busy, I was really tired and went to sleep right away.

Chapter 28

Thursday, October 26

More Visitors

The doctors reduced Joe's steroids to 55 mg. and, when his nurse tried to get a blood sample, she couldn't find a vein, and it took a couple of tries by a couple of people. He just hated all those pokes. He saw the normal doctors and therapists in the morning.

After his lunch, the corpsman helped Joe into the recliner chair while I went to get my lunch. I pushed him to the computer room when I returned. He had enough control of his hands to answer his own e-mails, so I rolled him to a computer then left him there while I ran back to his room to grab my food. I hurried in, picked up my salad and Pepsi, then turned to leave — and was surprised by a tall, handsome Marine coming toward me. It was Sgt. Major Estrada — the highest ranking enlisted man in the Marine Corps. While I had never met him, I knew that he had seen Joe twice — a few hours before I got to his room in Germany, then again with the Commandant a few days after we arrived at Bethesda. We both laughed when I nearly plowed into him as I hurried around the curtain.

Sgt. Major Estrada was pleased to hear that Joe was in the computer room and operating the computer on his own, he hadn't seen him since he was on life support in ICU, and was excited to hear of his progress. We spoke as if we were old friends, as we made our way to the computer room.

When we got there the Sgt. Major saw Joe immediately. I had moved the computer chair to the side to make room for the recliner chair that Joe was in, and Sgt. Major Estrada slid right into it. Joe glanced over, expecting that it was me coming back, and jumped back in shock. He recognized the Sgt. Major immediately, smiled real big, then shook his hand. The Sgt. Major was very personable and you would never guess that he outranked nearly everyone in the building. He spoke to Joe like an old friend, asking him how he was feeling and how he was progressing. It was easy to see that he had a big heart and was genuinely interested in his men.

He told Joe that he'd been back to Germany, visiting the patients at Landstuhl, and several people there had asked about him. I was surprised, with all the patients coming through the hospital, that they would remember one in particular. Perhaps it was because his story was so different from all the others. Sgt. Major Estrada said that one nurse, in particular, had asked him to send an e-mail, telling her how Joe was doing. He thought it was Sgt. Martinez. That name didn't sound familiar to me, but it was possible that I hadn't met her when I was there. He stayed for about 15 minutes, and wished Joe the best when he left — and he mentioned again that he'd be sending an e-mail to Landstuhl telling everyone of Joe's progress. His energy was invigorating and his visit encouraged both of us.

When we returned to Joe's room, the nurses were taking Brian to surgery to have a pain blocker inserted — I got the impression that it was something like a spinal block. My cell phone rang as they wheeled him out. It was Lou.

He told me about his business trip and promised to be home in a few days. He seemed to be getting homesick and I tried to go along with his story. I wasn't sure how much longer he would be content where he was.

Six members of the New York Police Department visited Joe that afternoon. They had all been near the twin towers when they fell in 2001. They told us that they visited Bethesda and Walter Reed two or three times a year to visit and encourage the patients. They thanked Joe for carrying on the fight against terrorism and gave him a shirt and cap. They were there about 15 minutes, and had such interesting stories, the time passed quickly. I was in awe of them; after what they had been through, to so selflessly visit the wounded. What a remarkable group of men.

While Joe was eating dinner, my friend Doris called from Lou's nursing home. She put him on the phone and he told me about his business trip, totally unaware that we'd talked just a couple of hours ago. Doris's mother-in-law also had Alzheimer's, and Doris had been the primary caregiver while her husband was in Iraq, so she knew how to talk to Lou. It was good to have someone like her there.

Soon, Brian came back but he was quiet and still groggy.

Dr. Montgomery came in for his nightly visit, Nurse Walling came by to say goodnight, I gave Joe a backrub, the nurses finished their last rounds, and by 9:00, Joe was ready to sleep. I gave him his IPOD and left for the Lodge.

Chapter 29

Friday Morning, October 27

Brian's Surgery & More Visitors

The day began on a positive note as Joe's steroids were reduced 50 mg. and the neurology team found that his feeling was down to T8. Joe had just started physical therapy when the corpsmen came to take Brian to surgery. He had become increasingly needy, constantly ringing the call button for help with something trivial, and a couple of the nurses had confided in me that he was driving them crazy. I suspected the pain killers he was on were causing his strange behavior, and I understood how his actions could irritate the nurses — especially when they were so short handed. We wished him well as they wheeled his bed out of the room.

Just as Brian left, Joe's first visitor arrived, three star general, General Sadler. We learned that he was from Alaska, had joined the Marines in 1972, and his mother and sister still lived in Fairbanks. I told him that I had spent 2 years in Fairbanks in the mid 70s and we had a nice little chat about the area. It was too bad that Brian was going to surgery; he would have liked to talk to the General too, as he grew up in Anchorage. The General talked to Joe for awhile and gave him one of his coins. I'd always thought that Generals would be aloof but I'd been pleasantly surprised to see how approachable they really were.

As soon as the General left, the Red team came in to examine Joe and talk about rehab. I got the feeling that they didn't know what else to do for him and would have liked to get rid of him, but I had learned that I had a great deal of say in that decision. It was somewhat up to me to decide when we would leave and where we would go and I'd decided to wait until I heard something impressive. So I told the Red team that I'd been talking to the social worker and we were looking into different places. They seem satisfied with that and continued on their rounds.

Joe's next visitors were 5th graders who had made get well cards for the patients. They didn't talk much and I was certain that it was an overwhelming experience for them to come to the hospital and see the wounded. They all wanted to shake his hand and have a personal contact with someone who'd been in the war. I was certain that it was an impressive experience for them.

The nurse checked Joe's blood sugar just before he ate, then brought in his insulin shot. It was easy to see that the feeling was coming back to his stomach. While he used to accept the shots without a flinch, he now took a deep breath and let out a manly "ouch".

Dr. Montgomery arrived at 12:15 with Dr. Collins and Laurie Duran from the Vaccine Health Center and we talked for some time. Dr. Collins told us that he had gotten an e-mail on Friday, October 6 from the hospital in Germany and immediately began doing research. He learned that Joe was already on a plane which would be landing in at Andrews Air Force Base in about two hours.

He called Dr. Montgomery and by the time the bus ambulance got to Bethesda Naval Hospital, he was there.

We talked about ADEM and how rare it is. We asked about the other 3 patients, who had gotten ADEM from smallpox vaccinations, and the doctors were evasive — patient privacy and all that — but they said enough for us to get the impression that the first two hadn't made it. The doctors said that they had learned from each patient and had applied what they'd learned to the next patient, so each one had done better than the last one. Dr. Collins did say that the last patient had been totally paralyzed and couldn't talk but had eventually gotten well enough to do a 60 Minutes interview. They didn't elaborate on that, but I got the feeling that the interview wasn't very favorable to the military. I made a mental note to try to find out about it.

Dr. Collins asked Joe what he remembered and he told them the whole story, from the first time he felt numbness in his legs until he fell asleep in the hospital in Balad. He told them how they had put him in a black bag and cut a hole in it for his head when they sent him to Balad in the helicopter. They had told him it would a cold trip and the bag would keep him warm. When he asked if it was a body bag, they said "No, it's just a plastic bag that will hold in your body heat." I had originally thought this was a hallucination, but it was the second time I'd heard the same story. Could it be true? Could he have left Fallujah in a body bag? We all chuckled at the irony.

Dr. Collins said that the doctors at the Vaccine Health Center would like to keep in contact with us and follow up on Joe's case, even for several years. They wanted to learn more and use their knowledge to help others who might be in a similar situation. We were under no obligation, of course, but Joe & I agreed that we should stay in touch and help others if we could. Laurie promised to contact us before we left Bethesda to get our phone numbers, e-mail addresses, etc. It was an informative visit; they had been with us for over half an hour, leaving just in time for the next flurry of activity: the nurse taking vitals, physical therapy, speech therapy, then Dr. Phun. He told us that Joe was his only patient, all the rest had checked out. He talked about reducing the amount of senna (stool softener) and possibly starting an iron pill next week. I got the feeling that we were a thorn in his side, if we had gone home he would have had no patients — and wouldn't have to come into the hospital at all. Too bad for him.

Chapter 30

Friday Afternoon, October 27
Brian's Meltdown

The real drama began when Brian came back from his skin graft surgery. He got into the room at 4:15, and pushed the call button for the nurse four times within the first 10 minutes. It was going to be a long night for the nurses.

I had told the nurses that I wanted to take Joe downstairs for the Friday night dinner in the executive dining room (my fourth dinner) and they had agreed that it would be a good outing for him. I asked them to start moving him into a wheelchair by 5:00 so we could get there by 6:00. It was only a 5 or 10 minute walk, but experience had shown that everything took a lot longer when we had to depend on help to get Joe ready. At 4:30, I asked the nurse to help me get him into the chair but before she could do anything, Brian called her over to his side of the room because he was having pain in his bladder. She told him that he had a catheter in and that was probably what was hurting him. He insisted that he needed to see a doctor and she went out to call him.

At 5:15, Brian's doctors came in and checked him for a hernia. It sounded rather painful from our side of the curtain and Joe & I both winced when Brian cried out. They decided that he was having bladder spasms and offered to give him medication for it. He asked if he could have the catheter removed and they agreed to send the nurse in to take care of it. Then they were gone.

Most of the time, Brian and Joe keep the curtain open so they could see and talk to each other. It helped to pass the time when they were bored, but when the doctors came in they always pulled the curtain shut to preserve privacy. There wasn't much privacy because the sounds weren't hampered at all. Many times, in his drug induced haze, Brian had attempted to talk to Joe's doctors as they examined him — like he needed to be consulted too. We always smiled, shook our heads, and ignored him. He responded by turning up the sound on his television — louder and louder — which really irritated the doctors.

The tables had been turned, Brian was being examined and we were on the other side of the curtain listening in. After the doctors left, time must have passed very slowly for Brian, and within one minute he began to talk about pulling the catheter out himself.

"Maybe I could just pull it out myself. It hurts SO BAD. I don't think I can stand it much longer. Where IS that nurse? They are so slow around here. I wish she would hurry up. Oh, it hurts SO BAD," he said.

Joe & I looked at each other, it was obvious that he was in pain but neither of us could help him at that point. We tried to wait patiently and quietly for the nurse. Then it happened.

"Joe, hey, Joe, are you over there?"

"Yeah, Brian, we're here"

"Oh, man, this hurts so bad. What should I do?"

We looked at each other again. What should he do? "Just hang in there, man, the nurse will be here any minute and she'll help you out," Joe said. Good answer, I thought.

"No, I don't think I can wait on her. She's too slow; she may not be here for an hour."

"No, I think you should wait, it won't be that long." Another good answer.

"Well, you have a catheter so you must know something about them, right?"

"Ummm, I guess so."

"Well, can't I just grab it and pull it out?"

"No, Brian, I wouldn't do that if I were you. Those things are held in place somehow, and I've heard they have to loosen the connection, or whatever. No, that probably wouldn't be a very good idea," he said.

"I think I'm going to do it. I'm just going to grab it and pull real hard. Don't you think that would work?"

Joe and I looked at each other again. "I don't think you better do that, Brian. I don't really know, but I've heard of people who've had those things pulled out and I've heard it's really painful." I said.

Brian tried again, "I'm in pain now! How much more could it hurt?"

"A lot," Joe and I said together. He was in such pain; I hoped he didn't get desperate enough to do it.

Just then, the nurse walked in the door — it had only been 10 minutes since the doctors had left the room — but it had been a L-O-N-G ten minutes!

"I'm so glad you're here. This hurts so bad, I was thinking of pulling it out myself," we heard Brian tell the nurse.

She just laughed and laughed. "You must be kidding me," she said, "These things are held in with a little ring that we fill with saline solution. We have to release the solution before we can pull them out. You might have pulled the whole end of your dinger off if you'd done that."

It wasn't really funny, but yet it was, and Joe & I both covered our mouths so Brian couldn't hear us laughing. It was also a great relief. In no time at all, the nurse had removed the catheter and brought Brian a urinal. He was no longer in pain and must have thanked her a hundred times. Now, maybe things could get back to normal.

I called over to the nurse and reminded her that we'd asked for a wheelchair two hours earlier and needed to be on our way downstairs within the next 30 minutes. She said she'd check on it but couldn't promise anything. It irritated me that I would ask for something that should be easily done and hours later, still be waiting. I didn't have long to fume because Dr. Montgomery walked in. He only stayed about 10 minutes and by the time he left, Brian was sound asleep.

I went out in the hall to wait for a wheelchair and while I was standing there, Cpl. Lopes came by. As I was talking him, one of the nurses came by and promised to get a wheelchair right away. Just seeing me talking to one of the Liaisons seemed to get things moving along, and it had worked again. I guess I had developed a reputation! Within minutes, there were 2 corpsmen in the room getting Joe ready to go.

While we were waiting, a lady walked over and joined our conversation. Her name was Helen and she was a volunteer with the Semper Fi Fund. She asked for my application form, which I got from Joe's room and gave to her. I still didn't know what the fund was all about, but I liked Helen instantly. As it turned out, the Semper Fi

Fund is a <u>wonderful</u> thing, and Helen remains a good friend to this day.

There was another Marine, just back from Iraq, in Room 06, and I had talked to his mother, Amanda, about the dinner earlier in the day. When she heard us talking in the hall, she came out and, decided to go to dinner with us. Since we didn't have time to wait on a wheelchair any longer, I asked the corpsmen to help Joe into the recliner. They lifted him into the recliner chair, and at 6:00 sharp, we left with Amanda for the executive dining room. It was my fourth meal, and the first time for Joe.

We were a little late for dinner, but the chefs were all happy to see us, as always. Most of the seats were full, but there were a couple of empty spots on the far side of the room. It took a bit of effort, but I finally got the recliner chair maneuvered around the room and we settled in. One of the chefs came over to say that they were serving chicken but only had one serving left. Since Joe and I are vegetarians, they gave the last of the chicken to Amanda, and it all worked out.

We saw several families that we knew, but they were all on the other side of the room. The family sitting nearest to us had just arrived that day and hadn't even seen their patient yet as he'd been taken to surgery as soon as he arrived from Germany. I was surprised to hear that he was in the Army and asked his wife why he hadn't gone to Walter Reed. She was also puzzled by that, but thought it might have been because of the nature of his head injury.

The dinner was nice — tomato soup, salad, mashed potatoes, asparagus and a brownie with ice cream. It was Joe's first "real meal" and he really enjoyed it. The two of us lingered in the dining room until everyone else was gone and the chefs had begun their clean up. They let us hang out and relax, and a couple of them even came over and chatted with us for awhile. We had been there for over an hour when we finally decided it was time to go back upstairs.

"You know, I missed a perfect opportunity to put a hurt on an officer today," Joe said.

"What do you mean?" I asked.

"Well, you know, you always want to mess with the person bossing you around. It's human instinct."

"Yes, I know."

"Well, if I had just told Brian to grab that tube and yank real hard…."

"That would have been evil!"

"Yeah, I know," he grinned, and we both laughed. It was good to see that he still had his sense of humor.

We went to the computer room and had just sat down at the computers when Mr. Johnson came in. I was surprised to see him as I knew his son had been transferred to a VA hospital earlier in the week.

He told me that they had taken his son, by ambulance, to the VA Hospital in Richmond, which took a couple of hours. He had ridden in the ambulance with him. There were a couple of older gentlemen also checking in, so the doctor grouped them together and talked to all of them. The doctor told them that they would be working with a therapist who would help them learn to cope with their disabilities. When asked about helping them to improve, he seemed shocked and said that wasn't their job. Then the doctor started working with Johnson's son and, within minutes, the boy was crying and begging his dad to help him. "Please don't let him touch me again, all he does is hurt me and he doesn't even try to keep from hurting me." When Johnson confronted the doctor, he was told that they weren't there to make his son feel better or get better, they were only there to show him how to live with his disability and if that hurt – so be it. He told me that it took everything he had to keep from punching that doctor in the face. How well I understood THAT feeling.

Johnson had decided NOT to leave his boy alone for even a minute, pulled out his cell phone and called his son's doctor at Bethesda. The doctor arranged to have him transferred back to Bethesda and even found the ambulance drivers who had transported them to Richmond. They had stopped for lunch and were just getting ready to leave, so it was easy for them to go back to the VA hospital and pick them up. They planned to spend the night at the Navy Lodge (he even got the same room), then fly home to Texas in the morning. They would stay there for 2 weeks, then return to Bethesda where a decision would be made for future care. I wished him well and he promised to look us up when he got back, but it would be the last time I would see him.

After Johnson left, we met two sets of parents who had just gotten in. Their sons were the two 1/24 Marines who had been injured by an IED explosion which had killed two others. We had heard of the incident and knew that they would be coming. They weren't there long when their boys were wheeled down the hall toward their rooms. They were about to see them for the first time and we wished them the best as they left to follow the hospital beds. It was easy to see the anguish in their faces.

Joe was very tired and ready to get back into his bed, but when the corpsman came to lift him, they discovered that the bed wasn't working properly. The head of the bed wouldn't raise. The nurse also looked at it, then they decided that it would have be sent for repairs. There was never a dull moment on the fifth floor.

The rooms on the 5th floor were not very large and it was hard to move the beds around without disturbing Brian, who was trying to sleep. His bed was between Joe's bed and the door, so we had to move all the other furniture (chairs, computer, etc.) and put the rails down on the bed to get it out the door. Even then, it barely fit. We managed to get the broken bed out and the nurse found an empty bed in Room 02 that worked. That was when the problem began.

The nurse was trying to hurry as she pushed the new bed into the room and Brian had stretched out a bit, trying to get comfortable. His good leg had stretched out past the edge of the mattress on the side facing the door and, as the nurse pushed the new bed into the room it hit the bottom of his foot. That jarred his entire body, including the leg he'd just had surgery on and he woke up with a blood-curdling scream! The nurse backed the bed up and tried again, hitting his leg a second time. Another blood-curdling scream!

By that time, I was yelling for her to stop and Brian (in his drug induced haze) was trying to pull his leg back onto the bed.

"What the hell are you doing?" he screamed.

"Just trying to move a new bed in. What's wrong?" she answered.

"Goddamnit, you're going to kill me," he said and moaned in a pitiful, painful way.

She apologized and told him that she hadn't seen his leg hanging over the side of the bed. I don't think it made him feel any better; it had been a VERY rude awakening for him.

We finally got Brian quieted down, got the bed in, moved the furniture back into position, and got Joe into the new bed. By the time I finished Joe's back and foot rub, Brian had quieted down and gone to sleep. Joe was sleepy too, so I gave him his IPOD, turned out the lights and shut their door. I was drained.

Just as I was turning to walk toward the elevators, Amanda came out of her son's room. She had had a good time at the dinner and seemed to enjoy talking with the other families but now she was livid! I stopped to talk to her. There had been a mix up in the kitchen, and her son didn't get a dinner tray. She had walked, in the rain, to McDonald's to get him a burger. It was one more example of why each patient needed someone there as an advocate. After awhile, she seemed to calm down and was ready to go back into her son's room, so we said our goodbyes.

I left the hospital at 10:30 and was glad that I had my umbrella with me as it was still raining. It was a gentle rain, a little cold, and I walked quickly to the Lodge. It was laundry day again and I finally slid into bed about 1 am.

Chapter 31

Saturday, October 28

Things Quiet Down

The usual doctors and therapists came in, and they had the nurses bend and tie off Joe's catheter to see if he could feel the pressure building up in his bladder. The neurology team talked about removing Joe's internal catheter and explained self-catheterization to him. Having the catheter out would reduce irritation to the bladder and reduce the chances of infection. While eating lunch, Joe's left leg began to twitch.

Brian was awake and hungry, and soon the drama began. He didn't like the breakfast they brought him and complained that they brought him graham crackers.

"What's wrong with graham crackers?" Joe asked.

"I hate graham crackers, I've always hated them," he answered.

I told him that I like graham crackers, especially dunked in milk. He thought that was disgusting and offered to give me the crackers he hadn't eaten at breakfast.

"Why didn't you just send them back with your tray?" Joe asked.

"I thought somebody might want them," he answered.

I thanked him for the offer, but declined the crackers, so he pushed the call button for the nurse. When she came in, he asked her to take the crackers away because "just looking at them makes me nauseated," and she took them away.

Since his surgery, Brian had been on a dilaudid drip, administering it himself by pushing a button. He thought there was something wrong with the machine because it wouldn't give him medicine every time he pushed the button, so he pushed the call button for the nurse again. She explained to him that he could only push the button and get the pain reliever every 6 minutes. If he pushed it before the 6 minutes was up, it wouldn't give him any medicine, so he started setting the alarm in his watch. That way, even if he fell asleep, he would be awakened by the alarm every 6 minutes so he could push the button. Again, I wondered if he was developing a resistance.

Joe turned on the TV and we watched the end of "Hook". We tried to be quiet so Brian could rest but we soon decided that he was his own worst enemy. He hadn't eaten much of his lunch and soon pushed the button for the nurse again. Joe and I couldn't believe how many times he was calling for the nurse; it seemed like every 5 minutes. The nurse came in again and asked him what he needed.

"I'm so hungry, do you think you could find something for me to eat?" he asked.

"The kitchen is probably closed by now but I could see if there's something in the pantry," she answered.

"Like what?"

"We usually have milk, juice, crackers, pudding, maybe even ice cream."

"No, none of that sounds good. Do you think you might have some graham crackers?" he asked.

Joe and I looked at each other in amazement.

"Yes," she said. "I could probably find some graham crackers. I'll go look."

"OK, thank you," he said and she left the room.

Joe and I were shocked, we were sure that he hated graham crackers. Oh, well, we went back to watching the movie. In a few minutes, we heard the door open and footsteps on the other side of the curtain. Followed very shortly by a blood-curdling scream! And another, softer scream.

"I'm sorry. I'm sorry. I didn't mean to frighten you." It was the same nurse.

"Oh, my God, you scared the HELL out of me," Brian croaked, obviously trying to catch his breath.

"I'm sorry, I was trying not to wake you and thought if I put them there you'd be sure to find them when you woke up," she panted. He had obviously scared her too.

"Oh, OK, that's OK. Just don't do it again, OK?"

"OK, no problem. Is there anything else I can do for you?" she asked.

"No, no thank you. That's enough," he answered.

She apologized again and went out, closing the door behind her.

By that time, Joe and I were about to suffocate ourselves, trying not to laugh.

"Holy shit," Brian said.

"What the hell was that?" Joe ventured.

"That stupid nurse about caused me to have a heart attack!" Brian answered. That was it, we couldn't hold it in any longer and we both burst out laughing.

"Sounded like you about gave her a heart attack too," I said.

"Did you see that?" Brian asked.

"No, the curtain is pulled, but we heard it," said Joe.

"She about scared me to death. I'm laying here, sound asleep and next thing I know, I open my eyes and there she is. I mean, right there, inches away from my face, laying something on my belly. What the hell?"

I laughed so hard I nearly wet myself. The way he described it was SO funny.

"And, what the hell, look what she put on me! Its graham crackers, I don't even like graham crackers. In fact, I hate graham crackers. Why, in God's name, did she scare the hell out of me to bring me something I hate?"

"Because you asked for them, man," answered Joe.

"No, I didn't."

"Oh, yes, you did, we heard you. We wondered what you were doing, because we thought you hated graham crackers. But we thought you knew what you were doing."

"Seriously?"

"Seriously."

"I must be losing my mind."

Truer words were never spoken. Just then his watch alarm went 'beep', we heard him push the drug button, and he was asleep again. Brian was more entertaining than the movie we were watching.

At 1:00, the corpsman came in to check Joe's vital signs and give him his medications. Joe told him that he had felt the pressure change in his bladder, and asked him to untie the catheter. It was a very good sign. The corpsman brought a wheelchair, lifted Joe into it, and we went to Subway so I could eat lunch.

While we were there, we met the owner, who was wearing a Marine Corps Marathon T-shirt. He told us that he had donated sandwiches the day before the Marathon for several years, and had taken 1400 sandwiches to the pre-run meal earlier in the day. He also told us that all of his businesses were on Marine bases and he owed his livelihood to the Marines. He was always glad to give back to the Marines. He asked Joe about his service and his illness, thanked him for serving, and then insisted that Joe try a cheese pizza. Needless to say, Joe liked it. I never got the gentleman's name, but he was nice as could be. He stopped to talk to Joe once again, as he was leaving, and wished us well.

It was a nice day, so we went outside and sat in the sun until the clouds started rolling in and it started getting chilly. We took our time, visiting the Marine Liaison office and checking e-mails in the computer room before returning to Joe's room. He enjoyed being out and being able to use a wheelchair made it so much easier for both of us.

That evening we had a visit from three MarineParents.com ladies. I had contacted them on October 1 when I was trying to find Joe in Iraq and while they weren't able to help me find him then, they had put him in their PAL program. The wounded Marines in the PAL program receive get well cards from many people and these cards would become an important part of Joe's recovery. Two of the visitors were named Tracy. Tracy Della Vecchia is the President and Founder of the organization, which is located in Columbia, MO, about 150 miles from Springfield. The other Tracey told us that her son, Neil had been wounded in Iraq and had been a patient on the 5th floor, exactly one year before. She told us that he was doing well and would be running in the Marine Corps Marathon the next day. After they left, Joe said, "Wouldn't it be something if I could run the Marathon this time next year?" I knew he was tough, but I realized then that he was a bit out of touch with reality. I was afraid that he really did have brain damage.

Later that evening, the nurse spilled a large amount of urine on the floor when she was emptying Joe's Foley bag. She left the room, saying that she would send someone from housekeeping to clean it up. About an hour later, having totally forgotten about it, I walked right into the puddle. I got some paper towels from the bathroom and cleaned it up myself. We never saw anyone from housekeeping. Brian thought we should complain, but I didn't think it was that important.

The rest of the evening was spent relaxing, watching TV and reading. We went through our normal evening rituals: foot & leg message, backrub, snack, and the nurse's visit to take vital signs and give evening medications. Brian was already asleep when I gave Joe his IPOD, turned out the lights, closed the door, and left for the Lodge.

CHAPTER 32

Sunday, October 29

Marine Corps Marathon & Lou's Escape

It was the day of the Marine Corps Marathon and it started out as a lovely day, a little cool, but a nice day for the runners. When I got to Joe's room, he had already seen some of the news coverage on TV. He was getting more and more interested in the race. I saw Amanda in the hall and she seemed to be having a good day too.

The nurses clamped off Joe's catheter again, the neurologists examined him and were pleased to see that his feeling was much lower on the left side of his torso. He was also moving his right leg more. His steroids were still at 50 mg a day and Dr. Fung talked about cutting back on his laxatives. He had physical therapy, was given his medications, then the corpsman got him ready and into a wheelchair. By 10:45, we were back in the computer room and Joe was checking his e-mail. It seemed like a normal Sunday.

Just before lunch, I got a disturbing call from Larry at the Rehab Center in Springfield where Lou had been a patient for the past 13 days. Next door to the Rehab Center was a church and the parking lot was full of cars since it was Sunday. Lou saw a car that he thought was his and tried to go out the front door but, of course, one of the staff stopped him. That made him angry and he went back into his room. The next thing they knew, he had kicked out the window screen, climbed out the window and was running toward the car. Since he had the alarm band on his arm, the staff was alerted and went out to get him. He was belligerent with the staff, telling them to leave him alone or he'd kick their asses. They considered that to be combative and called the police. They also called an ambulance and planned to transport him to St. John's Hospital for a mental evaluation. Larry said that he'd calmed down a bit, but he expected things to escalate again when the police and ambulance arrived. I thanked him for calling and asked him to keep me informed.

None of that surprised me, except for the jumping out the window. I had known about Lou's temper for some time, having been married to him for 26 years. He had never hit me, but I believe he came close a few times. I think he believed me when I told him that, if he ever hit me once, he'd never get a chance to do it again. At 74 years of age, he'd calmed down some, but apparently, not enough.

We ate lunch together in Joe's room, while watching the Marathon coverage on TV.

Grace called just as we were finishing lunch. She and my dad had decided to go to Springfield to check on Lou and had gotten to the nursing home just before the ambulance. What luck! It was good to hear that someone was there to help him through the situation. She said that he was at the end of the hall, surrounded by nursing home workers and two very large policemen when they walked in the door.

"Uh-oh," she said to my dad "I wonder what's going on here?" Just then Lou turned around, pointed at them and shouted, "There they are, they know me, they'll help me! Get them over here!" They were able to calm him down and convince him to get on the gurney when the ambulance arrived. The EMTs probably would have had to sedate him f my parents hadn't been there to calm him down. They met the ambulance at the hospital and were waiting with him in his room in the E.R. She agreed to call me back after they talked to a doctor and I told her how glad I was that they were there. It was hard for me to be so far away and unable to help Lou through the ravages of his disease.

Joe wanted to get out of the hospital and I need to go to the BX, so we asked for a wheelchair. It was so much easier since he was strong enough to sit in a wheelchair and it would be his first excursion away from the hospital building. He even took off the hospital gown and put on a shirt for the first time.

It took a bit of effort to get to the BX with a wheelchair. The short way had several stairs, so we had to go up the street, around a building, back around the back side of the building and down a steep driveway to the BX parking lot. Easy getting there, but I knew that coming back UP the hill would be harder. I think Joe enjoyed getting out and having something new to do as he helped me pick out the things we needed. We went to the Kodak machine, I inserted my camera memory stick, and we printed out some of the pictures I'd been taking. It was the first time I'd printed pictures since my trip had begun. While we were printing the pictures, one of Joe's ICU nurses came by. His name was John and he was doing some shopping with his wife. He hadn't seen Joe since he'd transferred out of ICU and they had a nice visit. He was excited to see Joe out of bed and wheeling around the base.

While we were in the BX, Grace called on my cell phone and told me that they were leaving the hospital to get something to eat.

Lou was calm and they thought he'd be OK while they were gone. She and my dad are both diabetics and I knew that they had to keep their blood sugar levels from dropping too low.

Joe and I made it back up the hill, around the backside of the building and started around the corner. That's when we saw the flock of Canada geese. There were about 100 of them and they had landed in the meadow next to the building while we were at the BX. We would get Canada geese in Missouri, as they migrated, and I knew that they would sometimes chase and bite people.

I'd heard that they bite pretty hard, so I told Joe, "If one of those things comes after me, I'm running and you'll be on your own."

"You can't do that; I'll roll down the hill into the street. If the geese don't get me first."

"I'll put the brakes on for you before I go," I said. He laughed nervously and he got lucky because none of the geese looked at me threateningly. Later he asked me if I would have really run off and left him — and, of course, I said "Heck, yeah!" Hee-hee!

When we got back to the hospital, we went to the computer room. There were usually several people in there, using the computers or watching TV. Lots of families would bring kids in, especially on weekends, to see a wounded dad. It was good to see the guys playing with their kids, but also sad. Many of the parents & wives would come in to relax while their Marine was getting a treatment or having surgery. There was usually someone to talk to, if you wanted to talk, or a quiet corner if you didn't. Everyone was very respectful of other people's privacy.

While there, we had some visitors, John & Diane, parents of a girl Joe knew at Missouri State. The delivered a box from Joe's fraternity, and we had a nice visit with them. It was nice to have visitors, and Joe was excited to find a couple of t-shirts, a small MSU football signed by his fraternity brothers, and lots of Halloween candy in the box!

During the time that we were visiting with Laura's parents, I got a couple of calls about Lou and left the room to talk. I wasn't sure how to approach Laura's parents with the information, having just met them and all, so I just excused myself each time my phone rang. My folks seemed to be stressing out, so I gave them my friend Julie's phone number. Julie worked as a nurse in town, and I was sure she could navigate the medical maze. They called her and she went right to the hospital to help them. The last time they called, they told me that St. John's was full but they had gotten a geriatric psychiatric bed for him at Doctor's Hospital (also in Springfield), where he would be kept for 72 hours observation. If everything worked out, he would then be sent to a nursing home with an Alzheimer's unit. Julie had done a good job.

After John and Diane left, we got Joe settled back in bed just in time for dinner. Grace called again to say that they were still at St. John's Hospital, waiting for an ambulance to take Lou to Doctor's Hospital. He had calmed down and wanted to talk to me. He told me that he had gotten into an argument with the guy who ran the hotel where he'd been staying, and they were taking him to another hotel. I told him that he needed to co-operate with the doctors and do what they told him. He agreed but only because he thought the new hotel would be nicer. Dad and Grace seemed very tired; it had been a long day for them but it seemed to finally be coming to an end.

Joe and I watched a special 60 Minutes report about the hospital in Balad. Joe didn't remember much about the hospital and was interested to see it. They also showed the inside of the hospital plane which Joe didn't remember at all as he had been in a coma for both flights. It was a good report.

The night nurse came in , took vital signs and give Joe his night medications; then Joe talked to Steven on the phone while I rubbed his feet & legs and put his cuffs and boots on. Soon after, the corpsman came in, got him ready for the night and propped a pillow behind him to force him to lie on his side. He had started to develop bedsores so they were trying to get him to lie in different positions. He complained that laying on his side made his back hurt, so I rubbed his back while he took phone calls from Andy and Steven. It was a busy night for phone calls. I asked Steven if he could come back for a few days, if I could arrange it. I was getting extremely tired and stressed out, and needed some rest and moral support. He agreed to come next weekend. Grace didn't call me back, they must have gotten Lou situated at Doctor's Hospital. I figured that no news was good news.

By 11:00, Joe was ready to sleep so I gave him his IPOD, turned out the lights and shut the door behind me. Brian was already asleep. I would learn later that Joe moved the pillow from behind his back and rolled onto his back before I even got out the front door. It was dark and cold and I walked quickly to the Lodge.

I was disappointed to find that there was no hot water for a shower. It was the fifth time there had been no hot water, I had had a tough day, and my patience was running thin. I crawled into bed, feeling grubby, and was soon sound asleep. I was exhausted.

Chapter 33

Monday, October 30

Long Distance Arrangements

I knew it was going to be a bad day when I woke to find that there was still no hot water. I stopped at the front desk to complain and was told that the boilers were scheduled to be replaced that week. It couldn't be soon enough for me, and I left still feeling grubby and grumpy. I was beginning to feel overwhelmed by the whole situation; it was hard to keep up with Joe's care, Lou's situation, arrangements on the home front, and still take care of myself. I could feel myself slipping into the darkness of despair, I didn't want to admit to depression, but I could feel it coming. I should have taken some Kava Kava.

As I was walking to the hospital, I ran into SSgt Perez and we talked about bringing Steven back to Bethesda for a week. He told me that there could be a way to use frequent flyer miles that had been donated to the Fisher House to cover the cost of the flight and promised to check into it when he got to the office. I was encouraged.

It was the beginning the 5th week of Joe's illness and he saw the normal doctors and therapists. SSgt Perez told me that Steven's travel had been approved and he would be working on the arrangements. It would be good to see him and I sure needed a break. Good news again, I was beginning to feel much better.

The corpsman brought Joe a razor, then stood by, just in case he cut himself. Even a small cut would have been dangerous given the amount of blood thinner he was taking. About the time he finished, a Marine Chaplain came in and gave him a very nice blanket. On one side, there was "USMC" in big letters and lots of Marine symbols and on the other side, a large picture of a tank with Marines all around it. The blanket was very soft and would become Joe's favorite. When Brian saw it, he commented on how nice it was and the Chaplain gave him one too. Brian was very proud to get his own blanket.

I called the nursing home where Lou had been and was told that he had been admitted to Doctor's Hospital. They put him in the Resolutions Unit, a lockdown area, where they could monitor him closely and evaluate his condition. She gave me the phone number and I called there to check on him. The nurse gave me a code to use when I called; the code was to protect his privacy. She told me that he had gone to a group therapy session and participated in the activities earlier in the day. He seemed to have gotten over his temper tantrum and was settling in well. I made sure she had my cell phone number before I hung up.

Cpl. Lopes came in to say that we should expect a visitor shortly; Billy Joel's brother-in-law was on the floor visiting the troops. We stayed for awhile, but Joe soon lost patience, he hadn't left the room all day and wanted to get out.

I took him to Taco Bell in the basement, then out to the circle drive to eat. We enjoyed the warm sun while we ate. We saw Mr.

Sharp and he was all alone. He'd had one or two of his kids with him for the past couple of weeks, but they were all back in school, and he seemed a bit lonesome. His Marine was in surgery, having his wounds washed out again. The doctors had to wash the wounds every other day to keep infections down and it was very hard on the boys and their families. The wash had to be done under general anesthesia because it was so painful. He hoped that his son would get out of ICU the next week. That was such good news. Soon he left for the smoking area and Joe and I went back upstairs.

When we got back to Joe's room, there was a plastic pumpkin in the window, full of Halloween candy. Brian said that Billy Joel's brother-in-law had left it. How ironic that we were out of the room the only time that a celebrity came to visit.

After dinner, one of the Marine Liaisons came in with an armful of mail for Joe. It was his first mail delivery and he would spend most of the evening reading it. All the mail had to go through an anthrax machine, so it took a long time to get things. Dr. Montgomery came in for his evening visit, stating that he was satisfied with Joe's progress, he might not do any more IVIG, and he thought we should start looking at places for rehab.

Dr. Miller came in to see Brian and we learned that he was not only a neurologist but also a Catholic priest. He closed the curtain and gave mass to Brian. When they were finished, he stopped to see how Joe was doing and seemed pleased to see him move his foot. Dr. Miller was an interesting person, and had become an encouragement to Joe. After he left, we completed our evening routine: foot and leg message, and putting boots and pumpers on. While he was probably moving around enough that the pumpers weren't necessary, we continued using them as added protection against blood clots. Joe always wore them when he was in bed.

We relaxed, reading the newspaper and Joe's mail, and watching Deal or No Deal on TV. Brian was asleep by the time I gave Joe his IPOD, turned out the lights, and left for the Lodge. The lukewarm shower felt amazingly good.

Chapter 34

Tuesday, October 31

Halloween

Early in the morning, they removed Joe's catheter and he was finally free of all tubes going into or out of his body. He was <u>very</u> pleased! He had a sponge bath, and was examined by a 4th year neurology student. The doctors had been bringing all their students to see him because his disease was so rare. I would hear them tell the students that they most likely would never see anyone with ADEM again.

I got a phone call from the social worker at Doctor's Hospital and he asked several questions about Lou and his medical history. He said Lou was doing well but the Alzheimer's was beginning to progress quite rapidly. They wanted to find a nursing home with a lock down Alzheimer's unit for him. I talked to Lou for a few minutes and he was pretty out of it. He told me that he'd been talking to Joe and they were thinking about coming to see me while I was in the hospital. I just went along with it, the doctors had told me that was the best way to handle it. He wouldn't even remember talking to me after he hung up the phone.

It was a normally busy morning and Joe tried to use the urinal a couple of times with no success. We made a trip to the computer room, and returned to his room just in time for lunch. He ate most of it, his appetite was getting better each day. While he was eating, the Red Team examined him, and talked about rehab again.

I picked up a fax from Doctor's Hospital and hurried to the galley, barely making it before they closed the doors I ate my lunch while filling out the forms and there were lots of pages to it. I faxed them back to the hospital on my way back to Joe's room., and talked to SSgt Perez about Steven's trip.

When I got to Joe's room, I was pleased to hear that he had been able to use the urinal. I was beginning to think they might have to put the catheter back in, so that was great news! He was able to go a second time — a total of 225 cc — I never thought I'd be so happy about pee.

It was still early when the Halloween activities began — different people coming around "reverse trick or treating" — giving away candy, instead of collecting it. There were so many different people, some in costume, some not, I couldn't keep track of them! Even some of the patients were walking around in costumes. We soon had more candy than anyone's teeth should be subjected to. But it was fun. Between that candy, the candy Billy Joel's brother-in-law brought, and the candy from Joe's fraternity, we could have supplied most of the 5th floor all by ourselves.

Soon, Joe was hungry again and I warmed up a burrito for him. While he was eating, the neurology team came in with 3 students and they all examined him. I went out in the hall during the exams and talked to one of the neurology doctors who had also stepped out of the room. I hadn't been real impressed with most of the neurology team docs, but I did take a liking to Dr. Rigler, so I asked her what she thought of Joe's case. She said that she was encouraged by his recent progress and felt that he had enough function to one day recover 100%. I asked her if that was overly optimistic, but she stuck to it, saying that he was progressing much faster than she had expected. It was good to hear.

Chapter 35

Brendon's Story

Brenden is a Marine who had had a bad reaction to the smallpox vaccination about a year earlier, and he visited with us for about two hours. He was 24 years old when we met him, and had spent the past 14 months in and out of the hospital — mostly at Walter Reed. His reaction had been mostly respiratory, not paralysis, like Joe. His symptoms began when he got to Kawait, and this is his story:

Brenden got the smallpox vaccination in May of 2005 and shipped out to Kuwait in June. Soon after arriving in Kuwait, he developed a rash and suffered from fatigue. The doctors thought that he was allergic to detergent and prescribed antihistamines and creams. Eventually, he began to have respiratory problems. He was sent to North Carolina where the doctors told him they didn't know what was happening, and offered to give him a medical discharge. He declined the discharge and began doing his own research on smallpox reactions, suspecting that to be the problem.

Brenden contacted the VHC at Walter Reed and they admitted him as a patient in August of 2005. When he was well enough to leave the hospital, he moved into the Mulagdo House (living quarters at Walter Reed, similar to the Fisher House at Bethesda) and continued to be treated as an out-patient. At one time, he was on 32 different medications, including high doses of prednisone. He continued to see an allergist, and take anti-histamines. He had stopped breathing several times and was lucky enough to be with people who could administer CPR until help could arrive each time. His legs would sometimes collapse and refuse to respond and he suffered from memory loss, chronic pain and migraines.

Brenden had been diagnosed with chronic fatigue syndrome, brain damage, and several other conditions. He was recently retired from the Marine Corps with a 60% disability. That made him eligible for a pension, full medical and dental benefits, and college tuition reimbursement. His plans were to live close to his medical support team at Walter Reed and attend college.

Brenden highly recommended Walter Reed as a rehab center for Joe. He was very satisfied with his treatment there, and was confident that he would continue to receive good treatment. He described the facilities and staff to us and it sounded like a good choice. It gave us something to think about.

Chapter 36

Halloween Night

Dr. Montgomery came in just before Brenden left and we all chatted for a few minutes. Dr. Montgomery seemed to know about Brenden but he didn't know the particulars of his case. We talked for a bit about the smallpox vaccination in general. We asked why the military gives it when there can be such life threatening reactions like Joe and Brenden's. The short answer is that smallpox is an extremely lethal disease and our government fears that our enemies could acquire some of the virus and use it as a weapon against our troops. Since the bad reactions involve a very small percentage of those getting the vaccination (less than 1%), they believe that it is worth the risk.

Dr. Montgomery and Brenden both left just as Joe's dinner came and, as he ate, we talked about Brenden and marveled at how lucky both of them had been to survive.

After dinner, Joe was able to urinate 100 cc on his own and then his nurse Margie brought in the bladder scan machine to see how much urine was left in his bladder. She ran the device over his abdomen, determined that the bladder wasn't empty enough and told him that he would have to straight cath. The nurses used the scanner each time he urinated to determine whether to have him straight cath or not. While he was doing that, I went to Subway for a sandwich for myself and a donut for Joe, then returned to his room to eat.

We relaxed, read the newspaper and magazines and watched TV. It was good to see the trick-or-treaters on the news, it seemed to bring some normalcy into our lives. Joe tried to use the urinal several times, but had no luck. The corpsmen got him into a wheelchair and we went to the computer room for awhile to check our e-mails.

I checked on the driving distance from Springfield to Washington DC, just in case Joe decided to stay at Walter Reed and I had to go back home. It was over 1000 miles, too far to drive. So I checked the airlines and found that a round trip ticket was $500, too expensive. I decided that I needed to have him closer to home so I could at least commute to see him on weekends. This could turn out to be a tough decision.

When Joe got tired we went back to his room and began our nightly ritual: foot, leg and back rubs and putting the boots and pumpers on. The nurse came in with nightly meds. Brian was already settled in for the night and watching the news as I gave Joe his IPOD, turned out the lights, shut the door and headed to the elevator. It was ten o'clock.

There was a little chill in the air as I walked up the hill toward the Navy Lodge. I knew that I had to do the laundry before going to sleep and was quite irritated to find that my key wouldn't work in my door. I went back to the elevators and up to the front desk to see what the problem was. I had to sign a form because my orders had been extended, then the clerk put the new code on my keys and send me on my way. When I got back to the room, neither key would work and I had to go back upstairs again. By the time I got the keys to work and got the laundry finished it was after midnight and I was exhausted. I went to sleep wondering how much longer I could keep up the pace.

Chapter 37

Wednesday, November 1 to Sunday, November 5
One Month

As I got ready to go to the hospital, I reflected on everything that had happened in the month since I had gotten that fateful telephone call from Iraq. I thought about everything that had happened in that short time, how our lives had been turned upside down. I thought about all the people that had come into our lives and were now such a big part of us; and all the people back home, holding down the fort.

Steven would return, spending three wonderful days, giving me time to recharge my energy sources, and Joe would continue to improve. He had more and more movement in his feet, and he learned to use a straight catheter to empty his bladder. The doctors continued to reduce his steroids every few days.

Meg and I talked every day and explored several different locations for rehab including VA facilities in Tampa, Minnesota, and Colorado. There were also VA facilities in St. Louis, Columbia and Kansas City — but I kept asking for something closer to home — and she finally agreed to check on a hospital in Springfield.

I called my friend Susie, whose husband was a prominent doctor in Springfield, specializing in hard to solve cases. He highly recommended St. John's Hospital in Springfield, which was good to hear. He told me that they used IVIG at St. John's, so we could get it there, if necessary.

Brian went for another surgery, did well, and was discharged from the hospital a few days after his baby went home. In true Marine fashion, he returned on the Marine Corps Birthday to celebrate with Joe.

We got Joe's medical records from Germany and Iraq and I was amazed to see that he really did leave Fallujah in a body bag. There it was, in black and white, under "method of transportation", a big check mark next to "body bag". And we thought it was a hallucination.

I met other parents, including Tony's mom. Tony was with Charlie Company and had been shot 6 times. His vest had stopped all but one bullet, which hit his hand. His mom said that he was recovering well.

By November 5, Joe could feel most of his body but the lower legs were still numb. He could move his right foot, toes and leg; but only the toes on the left leg.

Chapter 38

Monday, November 6 and Tuesday, November 7

Feeling Bad

It was Steven's last full day and when we got to Joe's room, we found him asleep with a pillow over his face. His ears were stuffy and his throat was sore, he'd had a hard time sleeping the night before, and the nurses thought he might have a virus.

Later, he got a phone call from Congressman Murtha. He wasn't our congressman, but he'd heard about Joe and wanted to encourage him, they talked for about 10 minutes. It was nice to have a call from someone is such a position. Joe also had a visit from some helicopter pilots, they were fun to talk to and gave each of us a patch. It lifted his spirits.

When Dr. Montgomery came in he said that he had conferred with Dr. Engler and they had decided to give another dose of IVIG. They had to wait 3 weeks between treatments, so the plan was to start it on Sunday. St. John's Hospital had accepted Joe and, if all went well, they would send us there on an Air Force medical plane after the IVIG treatment. He said that Dr. Engler was still in Guam but would be back in town soon and she wanted to meet Joe.

Steven left early the next morning and I was alone again.

That same day, we learned that Joe would be moved to another room. There were 8 new patients coming in from Iraq and they needed 4 rooms for them. The men coming in from Iraq had to be isolated from other patients until they tested negative for Acinebactor bacteria, and they couldn't put them into rooms where they might infect someone else. Since the surgical floor was nearly full, some of them would be put on the medical floor, so Joe would be moved into a room with another patient who had also tested negative.

We moved all of our things to the new room — Room 16 — on the same side of the hall, just past the nurse's station. His new roommate was a Marine Staff Sergeant who had been shot in the head in February and sent to Bethesda for treatment. They had cut out a section of his skull to allow for swelling of the brain. He had several surgeries and at some point, had experienced a stroke. They had sent him to the Tampa VA, but brought him back to Bethesda to replace the plate in his skull. He still had a trake tube in, and was on an airbed. The air pump was very loud and his bed and other equipment took up more than half the room. His mother was with him and she said that the doctors were planning to send him back to Tampa, but they weren't happy with his progress. He had regressed while he was at Bethesda and they weren't sure how much damage the stroke had caused. He had a wife and two little girls. His mother had been with him for the past 8 months and I knew it had to have been hard on her. He was a large man, and it was hard for the nurses to move him. The air bed kept turning him so he wouldn't develop bedsores.

After we got everything moved to the new room, Joe and I went to Main Street for lunch. On the way back, we stopped to hear a band that was playing near the emergency room entrance. As we were leaving, two guys in uniform stopped us, they had seen us walking and wanted to hear Joe's story. One of them was a Colonel who had had surgery on a disk in his back in August and he was at the hospital for a recheck. He told us that he was being deployed when he injured his back and felt bad that he hadn't been able to go overseas with his men. The injury happened the very day he was to leave. When they took him to the hospital, he asked the doctors to hurry up and fix him so he could get to the airport before his men left. Typical Marine! He told Joe that he'd never had the smallpox vaccination and Joe told him not to ever get one. Everyone we met had such interesting stories.

When Dr. Montgomery came in he said that he was thinking of moving the start of the IVIG treatment to Saturday. He told us that Dr. Engler had returned and we made plans to meet with her after the Marine Corps Birthday Party the next day.

That evening, Joe's face was red and he felt warm to the touch but his temperature was normal. He complained of a slight headache so the nurse gave him some Tylenol, which made him feel better.

Chapter 39

Wednesday, November 8
Marine Corps Birthday Party

It was a rainy day and I used the umbrella on my walk to the hospital. As I entered the lobby, I could see that they were setting up chairs and tables for the birthday party. Joe had already had physical therapy, a student nurse had given him a sponge bath, and he had on clean clothes. The physical therapist had tested his hand strength and it measured 35 pounds in both hands.

The nurses got Joe's roommate into the dreaded pink chair, and Joe into a wheelchair. It was around 11:00 when we went downstairs to the lobby for the birthday party. We found seats near the back, and Joe talked to several of the officers who were there talking to the patients. We watched as most of the patients from the fifth floor came in with their families. There were even two patients in their hospital beds. The Marine Corps Band was on the mezzanine above and behind us and when they began to play, at 11:30, the sound filtered down. They played for about 10 minutes before the Commandant arrived.

The birthday of the Marine Corps is a special time for all Marines, and to have the Commandant there was extra special. First the color guard posted the colors, then the Commandant spoke for about 10 minutes. It was a moving speech and Joe told me that an officer would read the same speech at all the other birthday parties around the country. When it was time for the cake cutting ceremony, they had the oldest (85 years old) and youngest (20 years old, born on December of 1986) Marines come forward. The youngest Marine was a patient and able to walk, but hooked up to an IV and he pulled his IV pole beside him. The Commandant cut the cake with the Marine sword and gave the first two pieces to the oldest and youngest Marines, then the color guard retired the colors and the Commandant thanked everyone for coming. The band members came downstairs and several of them shook Joe's hand. The Commandant and Sergeant Major came over to talk to Joe, and I took some pictures. They talked to most of the patients who had come downstairs for the ceremony and their photographer took lots of pictures.

We each had a piece of cake and some punch, then went back upstairs arriving just in time for our meeting with Dr. Montgomery and Dr. Engler. We all went into Meg's office where we were joined by three other doctors. We talked for quite awhile about the different options and then agreed upon a final plan.

The IVIG treatment would begin within 24 hours, with an infusion of 200 cc per hour, which is fast; but the doctors didn't think it would be too fast. Joe would be watched for adverse reactions for 48 hours, and if all went well, a medivac to Springfield would be requested. The doctors thought that he might need neuro-psychological testing for memory loss, an HCTH test and an EGD test after he got to Springfield. Everyone seemed content with the plan.

We saw the Commandant and Sergeant Major on our way back to Joe's room, they were visiting the patients who hadn't been able to go to the Birthday Party. Once again, I was impressed with their concern for the wounded.

When the neurology team did their rounds, Joe was able to raise his right leg slightly off the bed and roll his left leg from side to side. Corpsman Walling brought a Benadryl and put in an IV, and Dr. Fung brought in a discharge summary. We ate dinner, then settled in to watch TV and wait for the IVIG to arrive. We didn't wait long, as Nurse Carol brought it in at 6:10. She started it at 50 cc, then returned at 6:30 to increase it to 100. Meg brought in a form for the medivac request for me to complete.

Dr. Montgomery stopped by before he left the hospital and said that he was happy with the decisions that had been made at the meeting and also with Joe's progress. He didn't stay long.

At 7:30, the IVIG was increased to 150; at 8:00 it was increased to 175; and at 8:45, it was increased to 200. I watched TV with him and watched for adverse reactions. He seemed to be doing well and was getting sleepy, so we did the nightly rituals, and I left for the Navy Lodge at 10:30.

Chapter 40

Thursday, November 9

IVIG Treatment

It was sunny and warm and I hurried to the hospital to see how Joe had tolerated the IVIG treatment. The last bottle was nearly done and the nurse said he had done well overnight. By the time the IVIG finished, his temperature was 100.1, so they put several cold packs on him and his temperature started to come down. Dr. Phun ordered blood tests, a urine test and a chest x-ray — just in case Joe had an infection somewhere. The IVIG always seemed to send his temperature up so I wasn't concerned, but decided that it wouldn't hurt to check.

Over the next couple of hours, his temperature went up to 100.4. He didn't eat much of his lunch, which I attributed to the fever.

Several New York City firefighters with the Family & Friends for Freedom group came in to visit. A couple of them had been at ground zero on 9/11. They were very interesting and Joe enjoyed talking to them, even though he was still feeling bad. They thanked him for carrying on the fight and gave him a shirt. I felt bad that Joe wasn't feeling better while they were there.

After the firefighters left, and while Joe was sleeping, I went outside the hospital, enjoying the sunshine and 70 degree weather while I called dad & Grace. They were in Springfield and had just finished visiting Lou. He had recognized them, and had told them about the cars he was renting. He talked about the customers he'd dealt with and some of the employees. They said that he seemed happy in his make-believe world; and I was relieved to hear it.

As I sat there, watching traffic go by and enjoying the warmth of the sun, I wished that Joe felt well enough to get outside too. Andrew's mom came by with her dad, who was at the hospital to see Andrew. He seemed like a nice guy and I could tell that his presence was helpful to Diane. Just having someone to lean on, emotionally, was huge. As they went into the hospital, I saw Lt. Col. Workman come out the door and stand near a sign that said "Reserved for General". Another high ranking officer must have been on the way.

Joe's fever was gone and he was sleeping peacefully when I got back to his room. The IVIG always made him sleepy and feverish. I was confident that the IVIG was putting it's healing powers into action as I quietly left the room and went to the computer room. After an hour, I went back to his room and he was still sleeping, so I slipped out again. I surfed the internet for information about smallpox vaccination reactions and ADEM, and found some interesting sites.

Joe finally woke up at 5:30, just as his nurse came in to take his vital signs. She had been in several times during the afternoon, done her job quickly and quietly while he slept, and was pleased to see him awake and alert this time. He did a quick catheterization, finishing just as his dinner arrived. Someone had brought the mail and left it on his table, and he read it as he ate. There was a large envelope from Marine Parents with dozens of get well cards for him. He enjoyed each of them, and the mail-reading went on for hours. While he was reading, I warmed up my left over pasta and ate my dinner too.

The nurse came in at 7:30 and took Joe's vitals again. His blood pressure was 101/60 and his temperature was down to 99.3 — almost normal — it was good to hear. Dr. Montgomery came by, seemed pleased with Joe's progress, but didn't stay long. Steven called, talked to Joe for about 20 minutes, and he was visibly tired by the end of the conversation. It was easy to see that he was still feeling the effects of the IVIG. After the phone call, he complained of a headache (probably from the IVIG) and we asked for some Tylenol. Soon after the Tylenol took effect, he was ready to go back to sleep. I went through my normal, nighttime ritual, messaging his feet and legs, putting the pumpers on his calves and the boots on his feet, messaging his back, bringing him his toothbrush & toothpaste so he could brush his teeth, watching him take out his contacts, and giving him his IPOD and headphones. I turned out the lights and closed the door, hoping Joe would feel better in the morning. It was 11:00 as I left for the Navy Lodge.

Chapter 41

Friday, November 10

Marine Corps Birthday

Joe seemed to feel better, no fever and no headache, but he was still fatigued. I went to the computer room while he did a catheterization and met John and Kathy, students from the Naval Academy. They explained that they were out of school for Veteran's Day and had come to the hospital, bringing gifts, and hoping to see a few patients.

There was another mom in the room, and she took them to see her son, Justin, who had lost both legs in Iraq. As they left the room, she was telling them that Justin had been fitted for prosthetics that morning. He told the doctors that he had a request — he had always wanted to be 6'3", but was only 5'11" and he wanted to know if they could make him 6'3"! Once again, I was amazed at the spirit the injured Marines portrayed.

When the students returned, I took them to Joe's room. They were from Washington state and San Francisco, and Joe had a real nice visit with them. I was impressed with them, they had given up their holiday to visit the wounded. They gave him a stuffed animal, the Navy team mascot — a goat in Navy garb, which we sat on his television after they left.

Joe had a busy morning, with visits from the urology team then the Red team, who told us that the IV would be removed that day and the steroids would be reduced to 30 mg the next day. The nurse brought medications, the corpsman took another blood sample and removed the IV, and a wheelchair arrived just as Joe's lunch tray was delivered. He picked at it a little but was saving his appetite for something outside his hospital room. It was good to see him feeling better.

The Galley and Main Street were both closed because of the holiday, so we went to Subway for a sandwich. Since it was 75 degrees and sunny outside, we went out to wander around, eventually ending up at the big flagpole in front of the tower, where we watched as workers painted the pole. Joe was in a wonderful mood and we laughed and joked as we wandered around in the sunshine. The leaves on the trees had changed to beautiful fall colors and some leaves had begun to fall. A few trees had already lost all their leaves. There were lots of Canada geese in and around the ponds on the grounds and we watched them fly around for quite a while. I had my camera, and we took several pictures. Joe remarked that every day was like in the movie, Groundhog Day, an endless parade of the same things, day in and day out, with no end in sight. "I feel like, someday I'll get it right, and they'll let me leave," he said.

We finally went back upstairs to the computer room and were soon joined by Brian, Joe's first roommate. He had brought cupcakes, which he made himself, put candles in two of them, and he & Joe blew them out. It was their celebration of the Marine Corps Birthday. It was good to see him and, although he still walked with a limp, he said that he was healing up well. He said the baby cried a lot, but he was getting used to the commotion in the house.

I left Joe and Brian to talk, it was good for him to have a friend come to visit him. While I was gone, I called Doctor's Hospital on my cell phone and they told me that Lou wasn't feeling well. They had run some tests and, depending on what the tests showed, they would either treat him there or move him to the medical floor. They also talked about moving him to a nursing home, but hadn't found one with an empty bed yet.

After Brian left, we went back outside with Joe pushing the wheelchair himself. By the time we made it back to his room, he was really tired, glad to get back into bed with the corpsman's help, and was soon relaxing and reading a magazine. I took everything off his feet and he did a few of the exercises that the therapists had asked him to do. He was able to move and rotate his left leg from the hip, flex both ankles, and wriggle all his toes. There wasn't as much movement in the right leg, and the left side was definitely stronger.

Dr. Fung came in with travel papers for me to sign, and he examined Joe while I filled them out. He told us that tomorrow would be his last day on the 5th floor as he would be rotating out to another floor. He also told us that Joe was the only patient he had left. I got the impression that he felt he'd failed part of his job by not getting Joe out of the hospital before his rotation ended.

By 7:00, Joe was tired and ready to settle in for the night so we started our nightly routine of messaging feet & legs, putting pumpers on his calves, putting the boots on his feet and messaging his back. The nurse came in for final medications and vitals at 9:00 and I was relieved to see his temperature at 97.9. I helped him brush his teeth, take out his contacts, gave him his IPOD, turned off lights and left for Navy Lodge at 10:30. As I left the room, I noticed that his roommate was still awake and watching television. His treatment was over and he was just waiting for a medivac back to Tampa.

Chapter 42

Saturday, November 11

Taking Joe to the Navy Lodge

It was cloudy but warm as I walked to the hospital. Joe was asleep when I go there, so I plugged the headphones into his TV and watched it while eating the bagel I'd picked up at McDonald's. When he woke up, he felt the urge to urinate so I went to the computer room but it was crowded, and I went to the first floor lobby.

I saw Michael and his parents in the lobby and went over to talk to them. He was in the Army and I had met his wife at a Friday night dinner a couple of weeks earlier. I had talked to her and Michael's parents several times since then. As far as I could tell, he was the only Army soldier at Bethesda, and I'd decided that he must have come there instead of Walter Reed because of the nature of his head injury. I knew that the family was stationed in Alaska when his unit was activated to go to Iraq and the wife and kids had stayed behind there. They'd decided to move back to Texas after he was injured. Michael had just had his tour extended when his convoy hit an IED. Shrapnel went into his brain near the neck, then out the front near the hairline affecting three parts of his brain. His treatment was finished and they were waiting on a medivac to Tampa for rehab. The plan was for him to eventually come back to Bethesda for a cranial plate, then do rehab in Texas, near his parent's home.

I had seen Michael's mother and the kids several times in the lobby, they didn't like to take the kids to the 5th floor as they were afraid of the germs being brought back from Iraq. His mom usually watched the girls in the lobby while their mother went upstairs to see Michael. I learned that this was the first time the doctors had approved Michael to leave the floor and the first time he had seen his kids in over a year. Michael's wife had taken the youngest girl back to their room at the Fisher House and they were waiting for her to return. The other two children were playing and stopped to hug their dad from time to time. They seemed to be adjusting well to seeing him in a wheelchair with a helmet on his head. It was good to see him with his kids, more evidence that life really does go on.

I didn't know it then, but Michael and his family had met Bob Woodruff when he was at the hospital filming for the special about his Iraq injuries and I would see them on television soon. I made a couple of phone calls, as I watched the children playing, then went back to Joe's room.

Later, I took Joe outside in the wheelchair so he could enjoy the warm weather. We started walking up the hill, I showed him the little stream and the meadow where we'd seen the deer as we walked. Before I knew it, we were at the Navy Lodge, so I took him to see my room. The wheelchair was too wide to get past the TV, so he couldn't see the kitchen area, but he was able to see the rest of the room. He was interested to see where I had been staying. The trip back was downhill and much easier, and we went to the computer room where I looked for more information about ADEM.

It was 4:00 when we got back to Joe's room and the corpsman lifted him into bed. He needed to cath, so I went to the 3rd floor bathroom which was always much cleaner than the one on the 5th floor. I ran into a lady patient who was walking the halls looking for Lt. Dan, or rather the actor who played Lt. Dan in Forrest Gump. It seemed that the actor had been on 5 East earlier in the day, but he had already left. I also ran into Michael's mom and she was wearing an isolation gown. She was upset to hear that infectious disease hadn't cleared him yet, and she was very concerned that the kids could have been exposed to some nasty germs earlier in the day when he'd seen them. They'd been so careful.

Joe was disappointed when I told him that the Lt. Dan actor had been in the hospital, he would have liked to have met him. I ate dinner with him when his tray came, then we spent the rest of the evening watching TV and reading. It was a relaxing evening, interrupted only a few times by the nurses and corpsman. As the evening turned into night, I did my nighttime rituals and left for the Lodge at 10:30.

Chapter 43

Sunday, November 12

Relaxing Day

It was a rainy, windy day and I made good use of my sweatshirts and umbrella on the walk to the hospital. When I arrived, Joe had eaten his breakfast and the Red Team doctors were just leaving. They told me that they were going to print out his test results for us so we'd have them when we left.

Joe said that it felt like there was sand was in his urine, he had told his nurse and they were going to run a test. When the nurse and corpsman came to get the urine sample, I went to the computer room, returning a few minutes later to find Joe in the wheelchair.

Most of the corpsmen and physical therapists knew how to move Joe into the wheelchair, but there had been three occasions when the corpsmen had almost dropped him and I had to catch him! Once, he was being moved from the wheelchair to the bed and the corpsman had miscalculated how high the bed was. I had to jump forward, reaching over the bed, grabbing Joe around the waist and pulling him up onto the bed as he was falling. He ended up laying sideways on the bed with his bottom off the bed. The corpsman had to finish lifting him up onto the bed.

Another time, the corpsman misjudged the distance to the bed and started to set Joe down too soon. I had to reach around the wheelchair, grabbing him around the waist and holding him up until the corpsman could get a better grip on him and take another step toward the bed. The third time, the corpsman picked Joe up from the bed, then tried to get him to stand on his own while he turned him toward the wheelchair. Since Joe had no feeling in his legs, he immediately started to fall. I had to reach over the back of the wheelchair, grab him around the waist and hold him up until the corpsman could turn and lift him up onto the wheelchair. That was the scariest time as the corpsman almost fell right on top of him. Each time one of these things happened, it was with a new corpsman who had never worked with Joe and didn't seem to understand that he couldn't stand <u>at all.</u> I always watched closely when a new person came in to move him, and it always concerned me when I came into the room and he was already in the chair.

The physical therapist came in and helped Joe stretch his legs while sitting in the wheelchair. Soon after he left Joe had another visitor, a former Marine, who been out of the Corps for 2 years and worked for the government. He was a Morse Code and communication expert and his wife had been a Marine too. He said he came by the hospital from time to time to visit patients. They had a nice visit and when he left, he gave Joe a notebook and pen.

After he left, we went to Subway for lunch, then to the computer room, and I looked for information on ADEM again.

When we got back to Joe's room, I saw that housekeeping had left fresh sheets on his table, so I put them on his bed before the corpsman lifted him into it. The rest of the afternoon and evening were very quiet and we had a chance to relax and catch our breath. Joe's steroids had been reduced to 30 mg a day and the nurse came in early with his medications. Joe was tired and, by 8:30, our nightly rituals were done and he was ready to go to sleep. I went back to the Lodge and did laundry.

Chapter 44

Monday, November 13

Acinebactor

It was a cool, misty walk to the hospital and a quiet morning. The neurologists rated Joe's right foot a 4 on a 5 point scale. I wasn't sure exactly what that meant, but it sounded pretty good.

I called Doctor's Hospital and the nurse told me that Lou had had a reaction to one of his medications and was sleepy and more confused than normal. They thought he might have a blood clot in his leg and had done a dopler which turned out negative. His foot was bruised and swollen and they had done an x-ray of his foot and knee but didn't have the results yet. They were also planning to adjust his medications. Not good news.

Joe seemed tired all morning and continued to relax after lunch until Cross came to get him for physical therapy. He helped him into a wheelchair and took him across the hall to the physical therapy room where he showed him how to transfer from the wheelchair to a regular chair by himself. Joe's back was hurting, so Cross laid him on a table with a heating pad. Cross thought he'd been laying in one position too long, and he was feeling the soreness more as the paralysis relented. The nurses had been trying to get him to lay on his side for some time, but he hadn't been cooperating. While Joe was with Cross, I went to the post office and mailed a box home, and bought a tube for Joe's Commandant poster, to protect it on the trip home. I stopped at Main Street and bought 2 burritos for dinner and cereal for the next day's breakfast, then stopped at the computer room.

When I returned, Joe was in a wheelchair, wearing an isolation gown, and waiting for me at the door. He was visibly upset and told me that we would have to wear isolation gowns and change rooms as his urine had tested positive for acinebactor bacteria! He had been tested several times for acinebactor, always testing negative, and I was shocked to hear that he was now positive. Later, I would learn that the acinebactor bacteria can lie dormant for some time then suddenly become active. Because it was immune to most drugs, I knew that Joe would have to take strong anti-biotics to get rid of it. Reluctantly, I put on my isolation gown, left Joe in the computer room, and moved his things to his new room — Room 11.

Joe's new roommate was from the Washington D.C. area, and had been in a car wreck in Bahrain where he was stationed. He and his friend were on leave, and had rented a car. Another car pulled out from a side street and they hit it, flipping their car several times. The friend died from internal injuries and this young man lost his right leg. He had massive injuries to his left leg, had had several surgeries, and was afraid that he might lose it too. He also had head trauma. His was another injury that will be with him for the rest of his life.

Dr. Montgomery told us that we might have to stay at Bethesda until Joe tested negative for the bacteria, which could be up to two more weeks. Joe was very upset to hear that, again getting that

"Groundhog Day" feeling. I took him to Subway to calm him down, then we went to the basement and walked around the track twice. Joe pushed the wheelchair himself the first time around, trying to burn off steam, I suppose. We stayed out of the room for a long time, even watching TV in the computer room for about an hour. When we finally got back to Joe's room, he showed me how Cross had taught him to transfer from the wheelchair to a regular chair and I was impressed.

Joe was really tired, so I got him ready to sleep right away and left for the Lodge.

I had asked the nurses what I should be doing to keep from getting the acinebactor infection from Joe, and realized that I had been doing everything wrong. One of the things they told me was to wash our clothes separately until he tested negative, so I separated everything that I had washed the night before and re-washed it. That kept me busy for several hours and I finally got to sleep at 1 am.

Chapter 45

Tuesday, November 14

Our Last Day?

The walk to the hospital was sunny, there was a light breeze, and it was a warm day. When I got to the hospital and got my isolation gown on, I found Joe sleeping.

The neurologist came in to examine Joe's legs and found that the left leg was still weak but he could lift his knee off the bed. He was also able to lift the right knee off the bed and move his foot up to put his leg at a 45 degree angle. The Red Team told us that, if St. John's would accept Joe with the acinebactor infection, we could still leave as planned. They planned to culture his nostrils, underarms and groin for bacteria, and give an IV antibiotic for 10 to 14 days.

After lunch, Joe went with Cross to the physical therapy room again. While they were gone, I went to Main Street for lunch, to the computer room, and returned phone calls in the lobby. It seemed strange to have so much time to myself.

When we first got to Bethesda, I had seen a black man in a wheel chair several times, then didn't see him for awhile and thought he'd been discharged. I had seen him again a few days earlier, and saw him again from the lobby window — sitting outside in his wheelchair, smoking a cigarette in the courtyard area between the buildings. He looked up and saw me, and we waved to each other. I wondered what his story was. He always seemed to be smiling.

I went back upstairs, and found Joe in the computer room checking his e-mails. He wanted to go off the floor so I took him outside, enjoying the warm air and sunshine and talking about how the bacteria infection might keep us from leaving. Joe was upset, and I tried to calm him. We spent another hour in the computer room, finally getting Joe into bed just in time for his dinner tray.

Nurse Carol came in shortly and told us that we needed to be ready at 5:30 a.m. the next morning for our medivac flight. I was confused and asked her to page Dr. Montgomery; if anyone would know, it would be him.

Dr. Montgomery was close by and arrived about 10 minutes after he was paged. He had not heard of a discharge but was able to find out that, while there was a flight the next day, we were not on the list. Joe seemed to be disappointed, but I was glad to know what was going to happen, regardless. Another nurse told us that there was another medivac on Thursday and we could be on that one.

Corpsman Nav came in to start Joe's IV and blew it the first time! It was getting harder and harder to get his IVs started.

I left the room while Joe cathed, and ran into the black guy who had waved at me from the courtyard earlier. It turned out that he was a Sergeant with the 1/25 and he had been hurt in June. He lost his right leg below the knee and had been fitted with a prosthetic. His left leg was severely injured in the calf area and the doctors had taken a muscle from his stomach to replace the muscle in the calf. His leg had lots of scars from the surgeries. He had been at Bethesda for his surgeries, then to Walter Reed for rehab, and was back at Bethesda for another surgery to his right leg. He had a great attitude, a true warrior, ready for the next battle.

I also saw Debbie & Diane. They were both scheduled to go out on the medivac the next day — Debbie to Chicago and Diane to Minneapolis. They were both happy to be going home and I wished them well.

Joe's roommate had a visit from his dad, who lived nearby, so we watched TV quietly so they could visit. The IV antibiotic finally arrived at 10:30, took about 15 minutes to run, and Joe was half asleep by the time the nurse came back to unhook it.

I stopped at the Marine Liaison office before leaving the hospital and was again told that we were not leaving on the medivac the next day. But I had a strange feeling, as I walked up the hill, and decided to get everything ready so I could pack quickly when the time came, just in case I had a short notice. I organized my room, getting things ready to throw into a suitcase at a moment's notice, and finally crawled into bed at 1 am. Even though it was late and I was tired, I didn't sleep well. I tossed and turned, waking up again and again.

CHAPTER 46

Wednesday, November 15

Leaving Bethesda

The room phone rang at 2:00 am, waking me from a deep sleep. My first thought was that something had happened to Joe and I leaped for the receiver. The caller said that her name was Carolyn, and "If you can be ready by 5:30, we can have you on the medivac this morning; if not, the next one will be in a week. We've already told Josef and he's very excited about going home." My brain struggled to take it all in, but even as drowsy as I was, I knew that Joe would never forgive me if I didn't get up and get ready. So, after 40 nights at the Navy Lodge, I got my things together and checked out at 3:15 a.m., walking down the hill to the hospital for the last time while pulling my suitcases behind me. It was a cold walk but I was excited to be going home. At the hospital, I packed up the things in Joe's room and sent e-mails to everyone back home.

At 6:00, the medivac team put Joe on a stretcher and placed him on a gurney. They helped me with my suitcases and Joe's bag of medical supplies. I could see one team going into Michael's room, another team going into Joe's second roommate's room, and a third team gathering prescription bottles at the nurses station as we walked toward the elevators. It was a bittersweet experience to get on that elevator for the last time.

There was a lot of activity in the lobby and a blue hospital bus was parked in the circle drive. The medivac team rolled Joe's gurney near the statue and placed our bags on the floor beside him. Joe had complained of having a headache and one of the medivac women went upstairs, and returned with a Percocet for him.

They loaded our bags, then started putting the patients in the bus.

By 6:30, the bus was loaded, except for Joe's backpack, which I grabbed as I got in through the back door. The bus reminded me of an old school bus, with about 6 rows of seats at the front and room to carry 4 patients on litters in the back or 8 patients if they stacked them two high. There was room for the corpsmen to sit, and room for a limited amount of medical supplies. The patients were all on litters which were bolted to the walls on the outside and to chains hanging from the ceiling on the inside. There was room to walk down the middle of the bus, all the way from the front to the rear door. All but one patient was on the bus.

Joe was on the right side of the bus in the closest litter position to the front and I sat in the seat that was closest to him. The other parents were already in the seats in front of mine. They were surprised to see me, as we had parted just a few hours earlier thinking that Joe and I weren't leaving yet. I assured them that I was just as surprised to be there as they were to see me. Joe's headache had worsened, he asked for a cold rag for his forehead, and one of the women went back inside the hospital.

At 6:45, they brought the last patient out and put his litter and portable breathing machine on the bus. It took several minutes, but they finally got his wheelchair on too. The corpsman came back with ice packs for Joe and put one on his forehead. She told him that she had brought extra in case that one got too warm. He closed his eyes and seemed to be asleep. They took vitals on all the patients and double checked the prescription bag, counting each pill, for each patient.

At 7:00, the bus began to pull away from the building — just as one corpsman came running out of the hospital, yelling and waving at the bus! The driver stopped, the corpsman got on and everyone laughed at him because he almost got left behind. As we started moving again, they gave Joe his morning meds and another Percocet.

As we pulled out of the driveway and onto the street, I realized that I hadn't been in a moving vehicle for over 6 weeks — since that first weekend at the hospital. Being on the bus seemed oddly strange.

We passed through the front gate, turned right on the city street, and got one last look at the hospital and tower as we drove past. There were 5 patients on the bus: Joe, Andrew, David, Michael and Joe's second roommate. The family members were myself, Al & Diane, Debbie, and Michael's dad. There were 7 or 8 corpsman in the back watching over the patients. It was interesting to watch them as they got their IPODs out, and settled in for the ride. Only one person didn't have an IPOD, and I was struck by how popular they had become. I should've bought some IPOD stock. The bus turned onto a freeway onramp and we turned east, toward the rising sun. Joe appeared to be sleeping peacefully, letting the medicine work on his headache. The parents chatted excitedly, a new chapter was about to begin for all of us.

I thought about the people in the cars around us. Most of them were probably on their way to work, just another day in their busy lives. I wondered how many of them were thinking about us too, as they made their way around the big blue bus with the big red cross on the side. Did they know that this bus was carrying the heroes who had given so much to protect their freedoms, to keep their lives moving along? If they knew, would they care? The bus kept rolling along as we moved toward to our "new normal" lives.

When we got to the hospital at Andrews Air Force Base, they had all of us walk through a metal detector. They took our bags off the bus and ran them through a security machine. Then they separated us and we left the two patients who were going to Tampa there. Joe, David and Andrew were put back on the bus and we, the parents, followed. They took us directly to the runway where a plane with long metal ramps was waiting.

We had to take our carry-on bags and get on the airplane before they unloaded the patients. I checked on Joe one last time before I got off the bus, he appeared to be sleeping, nodding his head when I spoke to him but not opening his eyes. I could tell that the headache was still present.

As we walked up the ramps and entered the plane, I knew that my life would never be the same. We were going home, but our home had been changed forever.

We would spend the night at Scott Air Force Base, then fly on to Springfield the next day. An ambulance from St. John's Hospital met us at the airport and Joe was admitted directly to the rehab unit. My dad & step-mother were there to meet us and, a short time later, Lou was transferred from Doctor's Hospital to St. John's. We all went to the emergency room to see him and, although he looked bad and didn't recognize either of us, Joe was glad to get to see his dad. The Emergency Room doctor didn't think he needed to be in a hospital and he was sent to a nursing home with a lock-down Alzheimer's unit. One week later, on Thanksgiving Day, he passed away.

Chapter 47

November 16 thru December 3

Rehab

Joe began his rehab therapy and made unbelievable progress from the very first day. They began with physical therapy exercises in bed, teaching him how to move from bed to wheelchair. They taught him how to sit up, slide a board underneath his body, then slide along it into the seat of his wheelchair. It was difficult at first, but he soon mastered the technique. Next, they sat him on a portable toilet for a bowel movement, setting the stage for freedom from adult diapers. They introduced him to the Texas catheter, worn externally, which would free him from doing straight catheters every few hours. They adjusted his medications almost daily, in an attempt to find the perfect combination, giving him as much freedom and normalcy as possible. Such things that we take for granted had suddenly become very exciting achievements!

At his first physical therapy session, the therapist rated Joe's legs at 2 and -3 (on a 5 point scale). Joe's room had a combination shower/bathroom, a large room with a shower curtain right down the middle.

There were no raised areas and his occupational therapist rolled his wheelchair right into the shower area where there was a shower chair waiting. He transferred to the shower chair and enjoyed his first shower since leaving Iraq. I know that had to feel good.

Joe had been temporarily assigned to the 3/24 Weapons Company in Springfield, so they could better monitor his care, and Major Johnson and SSgt Segura came to see him that very first day. As the word got out that Joe was home, his friends started to arrive, and the local TV stations all came to do stories. I charged up the video camera and started taking videos of Joe's progress.

On his second day, his nurse came in with a special chair to weigh him. I had never seen a chair like it, and she explained that they used it for people who were unable to stand on a normal scale. Joe weighed 114 pounds. He had lost about 15 pounds since leaving for Iraq.

He found the computer room and went there as often as possible, and we left the unit and explored the hospital nearly every day.

On his third day in rehab, he stood up at the parallel bars, the first time he'd stood on his feet! He also sat on the toilet — another first.

On Day 4, he moved himself from the wheelchair to the bed with no assistance at all! He struggled a bit, but managed it all by himself. In afternoon physical therapy he walked along the parallel bars! It was the first time I'd seen him walk. He also used a tall walker, much more sturdy than a regular walker and tall enough for him to lean on. He was attached to a safety harness so he wouldn't fall.

On Day 5 he took his shower all by himself and used a different kind of walker in P.T. It seemed like he was doing something new every day. We both liked his rehab doctor, Dr. Bell, and she was happy with Joe's progress.

On Day 12, Joe went to Bass Pro Shops for his morning P.T. — his first official outing. He said that the trip went well, and he learned to use his wheelchair while shopping. In his afternoon Physical Therapy, they hooked up a stimulator to his left leg which stimulated the nerves in his thigh, sending periodic electric impulses into his muscles. I could see the muscles tighten up and relax with each impulse.

Major Johnson called to tell us that Joe's duffel bag had arrived from Iraq and then brought it to the hospital that night. His wife and son, Samuel, came with him. Joe was in the computer room, and we gave his wallet to little Samuel so he could have something special to give him, then we all went to find Joe. Samuel was SO excited to give Joe his wallet. We talked for a few minutes, then went back to the room.

It was like Christmas, Joe was so excited to get his stuff back — especially his laptop and his DVD collection. Everything was covered with a fine dust, normal for things coming out of that part of the world. We went through everything, checking the list that had been made when they packed it in Iraq. Everything seemed to be there except his "battlefield gear", and Major Johnson explained that they had kept it all in Iraq. It was just as well, he didn't need a helmet, bulletproof vest, and the like anyway. There were a lot of dirty clothes, so I sorted them out and took them home with me to wash. I can't describe how bad they smelled after being dirty and stuffed in a duffel bag for 2 months.

On Day 13, Joe was distracted as we prepared for Lou's funeral. His friend, Andy, took him to the hospital barber shop for a haircut. But that night, the rain changed to freezing rain, the electricity went off, and we had to postpone the funeral. When I went out to warm up the car, I found that the doors were frozen shut. I used a hair dryer to thaw the driver's door so I could open it, then I rearranged the garage enough to get the car in, leaving it there to thaw for several hours. Joe stayed at the hospital and did his normal therapies, even cooking pasta in occupational therapy. By the next day, there was 8" of snow on the ground.

On Day 14, Joe went on his second outing, this time to Lambert's Restaurant. I was totally jealous as Lambert's was our favorite eat-till-you-can't-eat-anymore restaurant. Lambert's had good food and the waiters would throw the rolls to you, literally. It was lots of fun! Three patients went, they all had a good time, and the food was great, as always.

Day 15 was a special day as Joe's steroids were reduced to 10 mg. But the big news was that Dr. Bell let him come home for a "trial run day". It was quite an exit as we took the wheelchair, walker and shower chair home with us. Andy met us at the house and helped me get the wheelchair up the stairs. It was obvious that I was in desperate need of a wheelchair ramp. I had rearranged the furniture so Joe could move around in his wheelchair and he was able to get into every room, except the bathrooms, where the doors were too narrow. His legs were strong enough for him to get out of the wheelchair at the bathroom door and maneuver around by using the walker and holding onto the counters. He didn't have to stand for long and he decided that he could cope with it. He was really happy to be home!

Joe worked on the computer for awhile, then we had lunch. I put the shower chair in the bathtub for him and he went in to try it out. He was in the bathroom for a long time, actually deciding to slide off the chair and soak in the bathtub. It was his first bath and he soaked for about an hour.

Dad & Grace arrived at 3:00 and were glad to see Joe at home. We all went to Zio's for dinner. The restaurant was crowded but we finally got a table and enjoyed a great dinner. Afterward, Joe wanted to drive past his fraternity house at MSU. It wasn't far from the hospital, and we were surprised to see several guys standing on the porch, even though it was very cold. It turned out that one of the guys had just left and about 4 others had come outside with him. As we pulled over to the curb, Joe yelled out the window at them. They all came over to talk to him and were excited to see that he was well enough to leave the hospital. None of them had jackets on, and soon they were shivering and ready to go back inside. It lifted Joe's spirits to see them.

I got Joe back to the hospital at 8:45, he got into bed and his nurse gave him his medications. He was very tired and I quickly got him ready to sleep, then left for home. Dad & Grace were already in bed when I got there, and it wasn't long before I was asleep too. The next day would be a long one.

CHAPTER 48

Monday, December 4

Lou's Funeral

It was still cold, but the roads were clear as I drove to church to set up for the funeral. I had made a collage of Lou's pictures which I set on an easel in the lobby. It included pictures from all stages of his life, at least since I had known him. We put a tablecloth on the table at the front of the church and sat the urn, flag, and two pictures on it. There was a picture of Lou alone and another picture of both of us with the two boys. They were older pictures, taken when he was still in good health.

Andy and Amanda were at the hospital when I got there and the two guys got into their dress blues. I hadn't seen Joe in his dress blues for over a year, and he looked very handsome. He and Andy together were stunning! I drove the car under the awning at the south entrance while Andy & Amanda pushed Joe to the door and helped him into the car.

Dad & Grace were waiting at church when we arrived at noon. We greeted our guests in the lobby area. They had closed down the entire Counseling Center at school and every counselor was there. Everett, our principal, also came. Several church members were there and some of our neighbors. Teri and 3 of the kids came in from Tulsa.

The ceremony was nice, then a much smaller group went to the cemetery. The memorial was held outside and the temperature was below freezing, but we all sat down, with the urn and flag on the table in front of us. The service was short, there was a 21 gun salute, and lastly, the flag was unfolded, refolded and handed to me. The cemetery director gave me the paperwork which included a map showing where the urn would be buried — after the ground thawed. We got back in our cars, turned the heaters on high and drove back to church where lunch had been prepared for us. It was nice to be able to relax and visit with our closest friends and relatives. All too soon, Teri had to leave for Tulsa so she could get home before it got dark and the roads froze over again.

I took Joe back to our house for a short time until it was time for him to go back to the hospital. He was obviously very tired, and settled, contentedly, into his bed. It had been a long and emotional day.

Chapter 49

December 8

Joe Comes Home!

Joe continued to improve dramatically, walking with arm crutches in physical therapy and going on a field trip to the mall. He learned how to open doors while sitting in a wheelchair, which he said was really hard. Three days after the funeral, he walked with two canes and even walked a short distance with just one cane! He was stronger and had better balance with each passing day.

Finally, after 69 days of hospitalization, 24 of them in rehab, Joe left the hospital as the cameraman from KY3 filmed — it was a red banner day!

We still didn't have a wheelchair ramp, so I had to pull Joe, in his wheelchair, up the three steps to the porch — then over the small rise at the threshold of the front door. "I hope I don't drop you," I said, half-joking. He chuckled, a little nervously — but we made it.

I called Steven with the good news, "Joe is home." This chapter was closed and another chapter in our lives was about to begin. It was exciting! Later that night, I paused in the doorway and watched as Joe slept, in his own bed, for the first time in his new life. Once again, I thanked God for the blessings in my life.

Chapter 50

Ups and Downs

The next few months would prove to be both exciting and challenging. We built the wheelchair ramp in the garage so Joe could get in and out on his own, no matter what the weather. The hospital sent a driver to get him to and from therapy each day and he began to make great progress.

About a week after coming home from the hospital, he had a surprise telephone call from Iraq — it was Adam Looney, his old roommate. They had become very close friends and they talked for quite awhile. I think it was good for both of them, they had both been so worried about each other. They had a bond that those of us who have not been to war will never know.

By Christmas, he could walk with only one forearm crutch and by New Years he could walk with no assistance of any kind. I went to therapy with him and videoed as often as I could. His tests showed improvement and he was excited to get on with his life.

Then, on January 12, 2007, Springfield was hit with a major ice storm. We had no electricity and no heat for 7 days and were forced to sleep wherever we could find a warm bed. There was major damage all around town, all the schools were closed for repairs, and we had damage to our trees, but not our house. As we moved around, staying in a different place each night, Joe began to get weaker and weaker, and by the end of the week he was confined to a wheelchair and unable to perform in physical therapy. It was hard to watch.

After our power was restored and we were able to return home, Joe began to improve, but after two weeks, he began to decline again; and on March 7 he was readmitted to the hospital. Dr. Bell and Dr. Zhia, his neurologist, agreed that he was having a relapse, another episode of de-mylenation. Only about 5% of ADEM patients have a second episode, so once again, he was breaking records! They decided to give another IVIG treatment.

As news of Joe's relapse spread, several people came to see him in the hospital and many others called me to check on him. Once again, the Marine Corps was there almost immediately, always ready to help in any way they could. But the best phone call of all came from Iraq — from his friend Adam again — his mom had told him that Joe was back in the hospital. I could have cried.

After a week on the neurology floor, and 5 days of IVIG infusions, Joe was well enough to move back to the rehab unit. He stayed there for another 10 days, as the doctors adjusted his medications and he worked in therapy every day. He remained weak and wheelchair-bound, using a cane only for short periods of time during therapy.

The day after he came home, he began running a low grade fever. We treated it with Tylenol and cold packs but by the following day, a Sunday, he awoke with a fever of 102.6 degrees. Reluctantly, we went to the emergency room.

They were busy and it was several hours before we finally made it to an examination room. Joe laid on the examination bed and turned on the TV, while I put his wheelchair in the corner and sat down to read the Sunday paper. He was asleep almost immediately.

We had been there for quite awhile, when the doctor came in. He was obviously not impressed with me, as he didn't acknowledge my presence at all. He merely glanced my direction and proceeded to tap Joe on the leg to wake him up. After the second or third attempt, Joe opened his eyes and the doctor introduced himself. Joe groaned and closed his eyes again. The doctor tapped his leg again and asked him to wake up and talk to him. He went over the nurse's notes — fever, aches, headache — then asked Joe if he'd had any childhood illnesses. "No," he croaked. I knew that he just wanted to be left alone so he could go back to sleep, as I watched the scene unfold from behind my paper.

"Is there anything else I need to know?" asked the doctor.

"No, I don't think so," Joe answered.

The doctor turned to leave. Now it was my turn. "You might want to tell him about the coma."

He looked at the clipboard again, "Coma? I didn't see anything here about a coma. Were you in a coma?"

"Yeah, but only for about a week," Joe said. I smiled.

"You might also want to tell him about the paralysis," I said.

The doctor looked back at Joe. "You were paralyzed?" he asked. "When was that?"

"It was after the coma," said Joe. "A few months ago, I think. It's in my file."

"That's his wheelchair over there in the corner," I told him.

"You're still paralyzed?" the doctor asked as he looked over at the wheelchair.

"Not totally," said Joe. I smiled again, wondering how much longer this could go on.

Still flipping through the papers on his clipboard, the doctor asked Joe if he knew what had caused the coma and paralysis.

"It was a reaction to a shot they gave me, smallpox, I think." He still wasn't fully awake.

The doctor felt that he was back in control again and he chuckled, "Oh, no, it couldn't have been smallpox, we haven't given that shot to people for 30 years." He smiled, that arrogant smile of someone who knows more than anyone else, but it was short lived.

"No, I'm sure it was smallpox. They gave it to me just before I left for Iraq."

"Iraq? You've been to Iraq? Are you in the military?" the doctor said as he began flipping through the clipboard again. Searching, I believe, for Joe's birth date.

I had heard enough, and began to speak as I folded up my newspaper and laid it on my lap. I was done with this guy who still refused to acknowledge my presence. "Yes, he's been to Iraq. He's in the Marine Corps and was given the smallpox vaccination just before he deployed in September of last year. His reaction caused complete paralysis and he was put on a ventilator. His official diagnosis is acute disseminated encephalomyelitis or ADEM for short. He was in military hospitals for almost 2 months, then here at St. John's for another month in the rehab unit. He still has problems with his legs as well as his bladder and should have a sizable chart here somewhere."

"Oh, well, I think I'll go see what I can find," he mumbled as he flew out the door.

"Hmmm," Joe muttered and went back to sleep.

I smiled and picked up my newspaper again — knowing that I had won the first round — that was fun.

Soon the doctor was back, making eye contact and talking directly to me as he let Joe sleep. Yessssss! He had found Joe's file and called Dr. Zhia. He was arranging for tests and had me go to the cafeteria to get Joe some food so he could take his medications. By the time Joe had eaten and taken his pills, they were ready to start the tests. They did a chest x-ray, blood test, urine test, strep test, and flu test — all of which were negative. The doctor decided that he had viral pharynitis and told me to take him home, give him Tylenol for the fever and call Dr. Zhia in the morning.

We finally made it home at 7:00 and I took his temperature again (100.1) and gave him more Tylenol. After eating dinner, Joe laid down on the couch and decided to stay there. So, I went to bed, leaving him on the couch. It had been a long day.

Chapter 51

Ambulance and Re-admittance to the Hospital

Joe continued to run a fever for the next three days, but his temperature would come down after taking Tylenol or ibuprofen, which we alternated every two hours. By Thursday, he was much worse; sweaty, cold, with vomiting and diarrhea. His temperature went as high as 104.0 and Tylenol and ice packs would only bring it down to 103.8. He wasn't able to get into the wheelchair and I knew I couldn't lift him, so I called 911 and requested an ambulance. While waiting for the ambulance, I called Dr. Bell and she agreed to arrange for direct admission. The ambulance arrived at 9:10, they quickly got Joe on the gurney and left for the hospital.

At the hospital, they started running tests right away: blood, urine and stool samples. They scheduled an MRI of the brain and started IV fluids. The doctors were suspicious of meningitis but soon ruled it out. They brought in a portable x-ray machine and took a chest x-ray. The nurse brought two Percocets and they tried to get him to eat some food. They gave him a Lovenox injection. Later that evening, he had the MRI.

It took 2 days to get Joe's temperature down, and the final diagnosis was dehydration and bladder infection. After 5 days, he was ready to go home again. Joe spent the next few weeks going to therapy every day, making some improvements, but he mostly used the wheelchair. Dr. Bell continued to adjust his muscle relaxers to help his legs work better, but the medicine seemed to make him even more tired. His legs didn't seem to be strong enough to support him, and he continued to lose weight. They tried putting braces on his legs during therapy, but he didn't do any better with them. Over the next few weeks, he continued to make slow progress.

Chapter 52

April 21

Marine Parents Conference

On April 21, we traveled to St. Louis for the Marine Parents Conference. It was at the Adams Mark Hotel, just across the street from the arch, and a 4 hour drive from Springfield. Joe was anxious to do something different and I hoped that the trip would boost his morale.

We met a lot of people at the conference, including Neil, whose mom had visited us when Joe was a patient at Bethesda. Neil's injuries were to his hands, he had nerve damage to his left hand, and had lost two fingers on his right hand. He told Joe that his left hand had a hole in the middle of it and, right after the injury, he could actually hold his hand in front of his face and see right through it! I remember thinking that he was fortunate they hadn't amputated.

Neil was a runner before his injury, watched the Marine Corps Marathon from his hospital room in 2005, and ran in the marathon in 2006 — when Joe a patient.

Neil told Joe that he was going to run in the Marine Corps Marathon again in 2007, and soon they were discussing how Joe could also be in it. They talked about racing wheelchairs, and Neil offered to push Joe if he couldn't make it. The others at the table joined in and plans began to take shape. I was amazed that his marathon dream, a dream hatched when he couldn't even roll himself over in bed, might actually come true.

We met a woman named Georgette, a gold star mom, who set down everything she was carrying (her arms were full), took off her glasses and gave Joe a great big bear hug. It was the first of many. Joe would say later that he'd never met anyone who hugged as much as Georgette. We would learn that Georgette and her husband, Roy, had a non-profit organization that they started after their only son was killed in Iraq. They call it The Heart of A Marine Foundation and by the end of the conference they had pledged to help Joe get a racing wheelchair or hand cycle for the Marathon!

We met Pat Kerr, the Veteran's Ombudsman for Missouri and, at one point we found ourselves in the elevator with her. She was also on the 10th floor, and on the way up, she started telling us about the excitement they'd had the night before. It seems that there was a guy in the street next to the hotel shooting a gun, he was acting crazy and the police finally had to shoot him, killing him. She told Joe that she watched the whole thing from her window on the 10th floor.

"I figured that I was safe enough, being on the 10th floor and all," she said.

"What?" Joe replied. "Why would you think that?"

"Well, I didn't think a bullet would make it all the way to the 10th floor. Would it?"

Joe stopped pushing his wheelchair, and Pat stopped too. "Are you kidding me?"

"Um, no, I mean, that's a long way isn't it?"

"Not for a bullet!"

Later that evening, Joe decided to have a little fun and told Pat that he'd looked out the window in his room, to see what kind of view he would have had if we'd been there the night before, and when he pulled the curtains back there was a bullet hole in the window! She fell for it — hook, line and sinker — and everybody had a big laugh. Joe was having a great time.

Saturday night dinner was a formal affair, so Joe put on his dress blues and I wore a long skirt. We met Major Corrado and it was good to put a face with the voice that I'd heard over the phone so many times since Joe's illness had begun. He invited us to Joe's unit's homecoming in Kansas City the next weekend. He said that while the family members would wait at the base, he would make arrangements for Joe to meet his buds at the airport. Joe was very excited.

General Christmas (retired) was the keynote speaker and he talked about the Marine Corps Museum in Virginia. He was instrumental in getting the museum built, and very excited about it. After his presentation, Tracy introduced Joe and Neil and was obviously surprised when Joe struggled to his feet. They got a standing ovation from the crowd!

One of the speakers was a guy named Russ, he had been in Iraq during the elections and had come into possession of some unused ballots. His goal was to give the ballots to the families of Marines who had been killed in action over there. There were three gold star families at the conference and, as he presented each of them with a ballot, there wasn't a dry eye in the room.

The trip was very inspiring and, as we left for home the next morning, I could tell that it had been good for Joe.

Chapter 53

April 23 to 27

Preparing for Homecoming

Joe had a tough week between the conference and homecoming, he was still unable to walk and still losing weight. His neurologist scheduled an MRI for the following week and ordered him to eat high calorie foods. She instructed me to watch for signs of infection, as his immune system continued to be very compromised.

Joe did poorly in therapy, took long naps, and even fell in the bathroom at home. The bright spot of his week was when he spoke to the Hometown Heroes group at Willard Junior High School. He was excited to be doing something different and the kids had put signs up all over the school that said "Welcome G.I. Joe". The kids were great and it boosted his morale. One of his high school teachers even came to hear him. He had a great time.

On Friday night, I took him to see a play at my school, "The Face on the Barroom Floor". It was a comedy and he laughed a lot. He was very excited about his unit's homecoming and started getting his uniform ready as soon as we go home.

Chapter 54

April 28

Homecoming!!

The big day finally arrived and we were anxious to get to Kansas City for the 24th Marines' homecoming! I had reserved a room at the Holiday Inn in Overland Park and we checked in just long enough for Joe to put on his cammies, then headed for the base in Belton. When we reached the road leading to the base, we were greeted by American flags on both sides of the road, it was exciting to see. As soon as we parked the car and got Joe's wheelchair out, Major Corrado came over to greet us, followed by several Marines who knew Joe. They were all excited to see him, and took him into the building. I wandered around a bit, talked to some of the other parents, and watched a video of the unit in Iraq, which was playing on a big screen.

Joe buddies helped him into a truck, placed his wheelchair in the back, and left for the airport. They were able to go all the way to the gate, where he sat in his wheelchair and waited for the returning Marines to step into the terminal. They were all surprised to see him and he had a great time greeting them. They all walked through the airport together and the people clapped as they went by. He said it was quite a scene. They got on the bus and began to drive toward the base. It must have been a sight to see, with the police motorcycles in front of the bus, and about 200 Freedom Riders on their motorcycles behind. There were so many motorcycles that they completely shut down traffic in the airport as they were leaving.

As they drove the 40 some miles to the base, they took up all three lanes of the freeway, driving at 40 to 45 miles per hour as the police stopped traffic entering at every on-ramp and the Freedom Riders blocked traffic behind them. It was all very exciting and, at one point, Major Wick told the bus driver to go faster as he wanted to get home "sometime today". Joe sat in the front seat with his friend, Sean and Major Wick and, at one point, Sean got out his cell phone and called his mom to tell her that he was sitting next to Joe. He was very excited, and so was she.

Joe said that, as they pulled off the freeway, there was a big sign on the overpass that said "Welcome Home 24th Marines". Traffic was backed up behind them as far as they could see and he said, "Now all those people know who to hate." Everyone on the bus thought it was funny. People were lined up along the road where we had seen the flags earlier, and the bus drove real slow so everyone could see them and wave.

Finally I saw the bus, pulling in slowly, making a wide turn, and coming to a stop about 40 feet away from the crowd. We had all been told not to rush the bus and everyone watched for "their Marine" to get off it. The police escorts stopped in front and the Patriot Riders gathered behind it. The door opened, one person got out, opened the hatch and pulled Joe's wheelchair out, then two guys lifted him down the stairs and sat him in the chair. The others followed in rapid succession and the crowd went wild as each family spotted "their Marine". Camcorders were rolling and cameras were clicking as everyone got that first shot. They all lined up, Major Wick called them to attention, told them when to be back on base, and dismissed them — he was fast, maybe a minute, probably less — and the crowd surged forward. I tried to film as much as possible as everyone was shaking hands, hugging, and kissing. I found Joe, gave him a big hug and welcomed him home, and we had a good laugh. We shook hands with as many of the Freedom Riders as we could, and thanked them for being there. Soon people started leaving. The guys were all anxious to get home. We stayed and talked for a long time, enjoying the excitement of it all.

We were hungry, so we went to Applebee's, and as soon as we were seated, a man came over to shake Joe's hand, thank him for fighting for his freedom, and welcome him home. The news came on while we were there, and we saw pictures of the bus on the TV over the bar. When we were ready to leave, our waitress told us that our bill had been taken care of by another diner. We didn't know who it was, and we marveled at the generosity of strangers. By the time we got back to our hotel, we were exhausted, fell into bed and were soon fast asleep.

The war was over for most of the men in Joe's unit, they would soon be taken off the active duty list and would return to the lives they led before the deployment. Most of them would remain "weekend warriors", completing their time in the reserves. A few of them would leave the Marine Corps and return to their civilian lives. Those who had made a career of the Marine Corps would go back to their stateside jobs. All of them would remember, sometimes with recurring nightmares in the middle of the night, their time in the war zone.

For Joe, the war will never end. Even though he was only "in country" for 9 days, he will always bear the physical reminders. Even though he saw minimal combat, he still looks closely at each piece of trash laying beside the road, always looking for that elusive IED that could do him in. Even though he never received a Purple Heart, he will always live with his injuries. Each day, for as long as he lives, he will take his prescriptions, and deal with the permanent disabilities as best he can. You see, my child is a fighter, a United States Marine in every sense of the word. He will give his best and perform at 110%. He will hide the hurt, the embarrassment, the pain. He will survive and he will thrive.

He is my hero.

Chapter 55

Smallpox Vaccination Facts

As Joe's illness progressed, I began to question our current smallpox vaccination policy. I started researching and the more I learned, the more questions I had. There don't seem to be statistics to show how many of our military personnel have experienced adverse reactions to the vaccinations they have been given. No statistics on illnesses or deaths.

I did find statistics that show that military deaths from illness totaled less than 200 per year from 1995 through 2002 (the year they began giving the smallpox vaccination again), and subsequent year deaths were 234 in 2003, 272 in 2004, 289 in 2005 and 247 in 2006 (#1). While there is no indication as to what illnesses caused these deaths, I believe that it is an interesting upward trend.

On December 1, 2003, the U S General Accounting Office prepared a report on the Smallpox Vaccination Program which stated that smallpox is a contagious disease that has no known cure and is fatal in about 30% of cases. The world has been free of naturally occurring smallpox since 1980. After vaccination a red, itchy bump forms within 2 to 4 days and indicates a "take". The vaccine uses live virus and the more serious adverse reactions are treated with vaccinia immune globulin (VIG) and the antiviral drug cidofovir. (#2)

The Center for Disease Control (CDC) quotes two studies from 1968 on their website. According to these studies, out of every million who are vaccinated against smallpox, 1,000 will experience an adverse reaction and most of these will be first time vacinees. Of these million, 14 to 52 will experience a life threatening illness and 1 or 2 will die. 1 in 83,000 will experience encephalitis. Recently, there seems to be an increase in those experiencing myopericarditis (inflammation of the heart), heart attack and angina. On the same website, the VAERS system, which tracks reported adverse reactions, has a listing of all reported events. Joe's VAERS number is 264693 (#3).

Routine vaccinations for smallpox in the United States ended in 1972. (#4).

The World Health Organization website states that, on May 8, 1980, "smallpox was declared to have been eradicated", "small stocks of the virus remained in secure laboratories", and "the risk of smallpox virus being used for terrorist purposes appears to be extremely low in most countries". During the smallpox eradication program, contacts vaccinated within four days of exposure "may be protected or at least develop less severe disease". (#5) This would lead one to believe that vaccinations could be administered _after_ exposure and still be effective.

Vaccinations were limited, due to a shortage of VIG between 1984 and 1990, and between 1990 and 2002 the DoD discontinued all smallpox vaccinations. (#2)

On December 13, 2002, the Department of Defense issued a News Release detailing a smallpox vaccination program "to protect the health and safety of military personnel". This statement went on to say that "smallpox is a serious infectious disease" and "vaccinating service members before an attack is the best way to ensure that our troops are protected.... if a smallpox outbreak occurs". More than a year after the 9-11 attacks, the DOD said that it feared smallpox could be used as a bioweapon. (#4)

The General Accounting Office describes the shipping of smallpox vaccines with computer chips to monitor temperature, and escorting shipments to ensure a tamper-free product. They also had a conference to educate those who would administer the program. A tri-fold brochure was developed, with web site and telephone contact information for those with adverse reactions. (#2)

In 2002 the CDC updated its guidelines for treating adverse reactions and designated the Army to be responsible for overseeing the program. That same year, a report questioning the accuracy of the information the DoD provided on the anthrax vaccination was issued. As of October 2003, the Army reported that 500,000 had been vaccinated for smallpox and 184 severe adverse reactions were reported. Two required treatment with VIG. The military was also monitoring several instances where a neurological reaction caused muscle weakness after vaccination. (#2)

The National Vaccine Information Center notes that there have been 106 life threatening events caused by smallpox vaccinations since 1962, with 98 of those in the past 10 years. (#6) Perhaps this would indicate that the current vaccines are more dangerous.

The first 5 months after vaccinations were re-instated (December 2002 thru May 2003), 450,293 people were vaccinated and .5% to 3.0% needed short term sick leave. There was one case of encephalitis and 37 cases of acute myopericarditis. All cases were reported to have recovered. (#7)

Of the 38,000 civilians who received the smallpox vacinnations in 2003, exactly 100 had serious adverse reactions. 95% were health workers. Of these 100, 85 required hospitalization, 2 suffered permanent disability and 10 experienced a life-threatening illness. There was 1 case of encephalitis and 2 cases were fatal. (#8)

According to the CDC "Adverse Reactions Following Smallpox Vaccination", for every one million first time vaccines, encephalitis or meningoencephalitis has been reported in 3 to 12 people. Of those, 15 to 25% will die and 25% will be left with permanent neurological problems. (#9)

Another report stated that 1,200 military personnel receiving vaccinations against biological agents from 2003 to 2005 developed "complex, in some cases debilitating, illnesses". This report included anthrax and smallpox vaccinations. The illnesses included "muscle and joint weakness and pain, chronic fatigue, intense migraines, cognitive problems, and severe diseases such as multiple sclerosis. Some of these have ended military careers" The report also stated that the numbers may not account for all serious illnesses because "military reporting on side effects is passive". (#10)

A DoD report issued in May of 2007 stated that over 1,200,000 military and civilian personnel were screened for vaccination in 2002 when President Bush directed the program to begin. Another 116,700 were medically exempted. Of the 1,200,000 vaccinations given 140 cases of myo-pericarditis, 16 cases of "ischemic" heart disease (heart attacks, artheroscierosis or angina), 61 cases of contact transfer of vaccinia virus, and 1 case of eczema vaccinatum were reported. Eight deaths were reviewed. (#11) While this DoD report concludes that the smallpox vaccination can be safely given, I believe that it is misleading, at best. This report doesn't mention any encephalitis events (I personally know of 5, including my son) or any respiratory events (as in Brenden's case).

In February 2008, the military began giving a new smallpox vaccine. Previously, the vaccine was grown on the skin of calves (Dryvax, made by Wyeth), now the new vaccine is grown in laboratory cell cultures (ACAM2000 made by Acambis) A new vaccine was approved by the US Food and Drug Administration in August 2007. The new vaccine is grown in lab cultures of African green monkey kidney cells and will allow "rapid and large-scale production.....with consistent product quality". According to Cynthia Smith, a DoD spokeswoman in Washington, the DoD has vaccinated more than 1.4 million military and contractor personnel since 2002 and currently gives about 15,000 smallpox vaccinations per month. Smallpox was eradicated from the world in the 1970s and the current program is predicated on the fear that terrorists could get their hands on virus stocks left over from the Soviet Union's biological weapons program. Only two countries are known to have virus, which is stored for research in one lab in the United States and one lab in the Soviet Union. This same article states that myopericarditis (inflammation of the heart muscle and lining) occurs in about 1 in 175 first time smallpox vaccinees but doesn't report a number for encephalitis. It also states that the new vaccine has a shorter shelf life — 30 days versus 90 days and the Department of Health and Human Services had already received 192.5 million doses. With the new vaccine, each person vaccinated must receive a medication guide. (#12)

The U. S. Defense Department reports show that in fiscal year 2008, nearly 185,000 joined the Army, Navy, Marine Corps and Air Force. Another 100,000 joined the reserves. (#13) If most of these troops are vaccinated, and the statistics from the CDC remain the same, we can expect 4 to 13 people EACH YEAR to have a life threatening reaction and one person to die from the vaccination. If we continue at current recruiting levels, we can expect to see the same scenario each year.

While there are many sites on the internet, citing different statistics, some seem to be more credible than others, and I have tried to cite the most credible ones here. I found that at www.thinktwice.com they claim that 12 to 14,000 reports of adverse reactions to vaccinations are reported each year, and 90% of doctors do not report. If this is true, we have a situation of epidemic proportions.

On August 15, 2008, the Huffington Post printed an article by David Kirby, who seems to have done a lot of research. He states that the DoD reports up to 2%, or up to 48,000 service members may have sustained "serious" adverse vaccine reactions, including disability and death. He quotes his source as stating that "multiple vaccines" or "drugs + vaccines" are the possible cause. (#14)

In an attempt to verify David Kirby's figures, I located a Vaccine Healthcare Centers Network power point which confirmed that one to two percent, or 24,000 to 48,000 service members had reported adverse vaccine side effects. It lists multiple vaccines and drugs + vaccines. It also states approximately 1.1 million have been vaccinated with two "possible" deaths related to myopericarditis. There is a "slow process of in depth causality assessments" due to the labor intensive reviews and a major challenge is "medical school…training is limited beyond vaccine schedules". (#15)

One young Marine, age 20, from Ohio, received a shot in November of 2005. Three weeks later, his kidneys were failing and his body was so swollen that it left stretch marks. The military refused to share information with his civilian doctors, and the shot in question was not listed in his military records. Eleven months later, his medical records sudden showed that the mystery shot was a flu vaccine. Meanwhile, this young man's kidneys failed and he was put on a waiting list for a transplant. An unidentified military health officer stated that "This is the worst cover-up in the history of the military", and "when the issue...of the use of the vaccine comes out...it will make the Walter Reed scandal pale in comparison". This is another strong, healthy, young man who has been medically discharged from the Corps, and is destined to live a life that revolves around his disabilities. (#16)

CNN reported, on January 31, 2003, that two servicemen had displayed "noteworthy" reactions to the smallpox vaccination. One was admitted to a military hospital overseas with encephalitis and the other developed a rash with pus-filled blisters. Both reactions occurred 8 to 10 days after their vaccination. (#17)

A CIDRAP report dated June 26, 2006 states that military physicians had determined that a combination of smallpox and flu vaccines "may have caused" the death of a young soldier at Fort Bragg, N. C. in 2005. Medical personnel also linked a combination of vaccines to the death of another Army soldier in 2003. This soldier's death certificate lists "diffuse alveolar damage" and pericarditis as the cause of death. This report also states that the DoD has investigated a total of eight deaths due to disease after smallpox vaccination. (#18)

At least one member of Congress has taken notice, as I have found a letter written by Carolyn B. Maloney, from the 14th District of New York. This letter was written on September 16, 2008 to Col. Engler of the Vaccine Healthcare Center, and Ms. Maloney requests more information based on the VHC power point. (#19) We have also heard from Congresswoman Claire McCaskill, who is our representative from Missouri

On October 24, 2002, CBS News reported that the Bush administration was preparing to ask Congress to consider how to compensate people who were injured or killed by the vaccine itself. However, the options discussed would be to protect medical workers who administered the vaccinations and civilians who received them, but there was no consideration for those in the military who receive the vaccines. (#20)

The Smallpox Emergency Personnel Protection Act of 2003 authorized the Secretary of Health and Human Services to establish the Smallpox Vaccine Injury Compensation Program and $42 million was set aside for those who were eligible. Members of the military are not eligible. (#21) The purpose of this fund is to assist those who are harmed by vaccines with such expenses as building wheelchair ramps, transportation to and from physical therapy, and widening doorways in the home.

The military provides TSGLI insurance for those serving in war zones, and Joe paid into this fund when he was deployed in Iraq. This fund is there to help with similar expenses as stated in the above paragraph; however, Joe's claim was denied as his was not considered a "traumatic event", even though his illness met two of the three included illnesses. In November of 2008, the TSGLI rules were changed and now absolutely no illnesses are covered, retroactively to a date before the military re-instated the smallpox vaccination program.

It appears that those with vaccine reactions during military service have fallen into a "no man's land" where they are not covered by the compensation funds set up for civilians nor are they covered by the military compensation fund. It's a no-win situation for those injured by vaccinations, and the vaccine manufacturers have no liabilities whatsoever.

Along these same lines, on June 15, 2007, an article written by Tom Philpott appeared on www.military.com. In this article

Mr. Philpott examines a congressional study which concludes that "VA disability pay set too low for many war wounded". This study examined disability pay for the youngest war wounded and concluded that it falls several thousand dollars (each year) short of what is needed to stay even with peers. (#22)

I have come across several young people in the military who became sick after a vaccination but the military didn't attribute the illness to the vaccination. These families have told me that, even if the doctors believe the illness was probably caused by a vaccination, they list only the resulting illness in the records because they can't be 100% sure that the vaccination was the culprit. If this is true, it may be impossible to determine how many illnesses — and deaths — may be caused by vaccinations. This type of reporting would also affect the number of adverse reactions reported (and tracked) by the DoD, causing the records to show fewer military personnel suffering from vaccine reactions. I have also heard from military members who were given several shots at once — a virtual cocktail of vaccinations — making it impossible to determine which vaccination or combination of vaccinations caused the reaction. These cases also seem to be reported as an illness due to respiratory disorder, muscle weakness, etc., not an adverse reaction.

In my son's case, he was ordered to report to medical and get the smallpox vaccination, was not told what symptoms to watch for or given the trifold brochure mentioned in the GAO Report. (#2) When his symptoms began, he had already been sent to a war zone and the medic assigned to his unit did not recognize that he was having an adverse reaction. When the doctors at Balad realized what was happening, they only had one method available to treat him, and when that failed, they could only try to keep him alive long enough to get to the United States for the second method of treatment. If he had

First One Home

been kept in the U.S. until after the window for adverse reactions had passed (10 - 14 days), he could have been treated sooner and probably had fewer life-changing medical issues.

It is disturbing to me that the DoD report of May 2007 (#11) does not list <u>any</u> encephalitis (like Joe's) or respiratory (like Brenden's) events, even though both young men have "smallpox vaccination reaction" noted multiple times in their military medical records, both have VAERS records with the CDC, and both are registered with the Vaccine Health Center at Walter Reed. It makes me wonder how many others have been left off — and how widespread these reactions really are.

For those with financial minds, the question must be asked: How much does this cost the military and taxpayers? I don't think I can wrap my mind around it, but here are the facts. If most new recruits are vaccinated (some are medically exempted), our military gives around a quarter of a million vaccinations each year and the cost of the vaccine itself plus the medical staff must be calculated. According to CDC estimates, around 250 people per year will require medical treatment and time off work, this must be calculated and added in. Approximately 13 people will have life threatening reactions which will require further hospitalization, rehabilitation, etc.

In Joe's case, he was hospitalized for almost 3 months and has a medical record of over 900 pages for this time period. He received 4 different IVIG treatments, numerous CAT scans, MRI's, blood tests, bladder function tests, etc. After discharge from the hospital, he had a full year of out patient physical therapy. He continues to see several different doctors and takes 5 different prescriptions each day. We are told that his medical issues will continue for the rest of his life. He will soon be medically discharged and will receive a check each month, based on his percentage of disability, for the rest of his life. How much will this cost the taxpayers? A lot. Now multiply that by possibly 13 others EACH YEAR. It must be an astronomical figure.

How much has this cost my son? He will never be able to do the things he used to enjoy: backpacking, hiking, bowling, rock climbing. He can't climb ladders, mow the lawn, change a tire, chop wood, walk to the store, stand in long lines, or walk around an amusement park. He can no longer be a Marine. Through the Voc-Rehab program, the military will send him to college and, hopefully, he will someday have a career and be a taxpayer himself again. This illness has cost him a lot.

I believe that the military could save some of these young men and women with a few changes in policy. If they would give no more than one or two vaccinations at a time, then wait through the 10 to 14 day period when most adverse reactions occur, symptoms could be treated sooner and more appropriately (they would know which vaccination caused the reaction). If they would wait until the 10 to 14 day period had passed before shipping troops to a war zone, adverse reactions could be treated sooner and there would be fewer lasting medical problems. If the medical personnel were better educated in this area, they could recognize adverse reactions sooner and treatment could start sooner. If all the young servicemen and women who are now experiencing reactions from multiple vaccines were not made ill and medically discharged, they could be productive members of the military.

Lastly, there is the question of why all childhood vaccinations need to be redone every few years in the military. This is not done in the civilian world.

Footnotes:

- # 1: Defense Manpower Data Center, Statistical Information Analysis Division; Table 5
- # 2: U.S. General Accounting Office Report to Committee on Governmental Affairs, December 1, 2003
- # 3: cdc.gov
- # 4: U.S. Department of Defense News Release No. 634-02
- # 5: http://www.who.itn/vaccines/en/smallpox.shtml
- # 6: National Vaccine Information Center
- # 7: J D Grabenstein, MD; U S Army Medical Command
- # 8: CIDRAP News; University of Minnesota, December 14, 2005
- # 9: cdc.gov
- # 10: Global Security Newswire, May 6, 2005
- # 11: DoD Smallpox Vaccination Program; Safety Summary; May 17, 2007
- # 12: CIDRAP News; University of Minnesota, February 8, 2008
- # 13: www.defenselink.mil
- # 14: "US Department of Defense: 1-2% of individuals may experience severe vaccine effects that 'could result' in disability or death"; Huffington Post 8-15-08
- # 15: Vaccine Healthcare Centers Network powerpoint
- # 16: http://www.wlwt.com/print/13271378detail.html
- # 17: www.cnn.com/2003/HEALTH/01/31/troops.smallpox/index.htm
- # 18: http://cidrapbusiness.net/cidrap/content/bt/smallpox/news/jun2606soldier
- # 19: Carolyn B. Maloney letter to Col. Reneta Engler of the VHC, dated 9-16-08
- # 20: CBS News; Limiting Smallpox Lawsuits, Oct. 24, 2002
- # 21: HRSA Smallpox Vaccine Injury Compensation Program
- # 22: War Wounded Underpaid by Tom Philpott; June 15, 2007

Postscript

It has been over two years since Joe first felt the numbness in his legs and our lives have taken on a "new normal". Time has relentlessly marched on and Joe is now 23 years old. Physically, he has continued to improve, surpassing every milestone that his doctors have set for him. Each step of the way, they caution that this may be as good as it gets — or he could revert back, even back to the point of total paralysis. The disease that was triggered by the smallpox vaccination is extremely rare, and long term survival is even more rare. Most doctors have never heard of ADEM, and the ones that have say that there aren't enough cases to predict what the future could hold.

After our trip to the Maine Parents Conference, the Heart of A Marine Foundation ordered a custom made hand cycle for Joe and he began training with it in August of 2007. I began training too and became fairly good at walking. We have been in some local races but the most exciting race has been the Marine Corps Marathon in Washington D.C. In October 2007, we raced on the Marine Parents Team. Steven met us there and we spent several days together, just our little family, in our "new normal" life, pushing Joe in his wheelchair, and sightseeing around the city. On race day, Joe raced the entire 26.2 miles on his hand cycle, finishing in the middle of the pack of 42 hand cyclists. Steven jumped on and off the Metro, getting pictures of Joe along the way, then meeting him at the finish line. I ran/walked the 10K, crossing the same finish line about 20 minutes after Joe. It was exhausting, but SO exciting!

We met Justin on that trip to Washington DC, a young Marine who also had a bad reaction to vaccinations. He had just graduated from college and started officer's training school when they gave him 7 shots in one day. He said he didn't know what they all were, but he did know that he did NOT get the smallpox vaccination. Four days later, he had weakness to one side of his body, headaches, and fluid on one side of his brain. At first, the doctors thought he was having a stroke. He was still having problems with short term memory and comprehension and his future with the Marine Corps looked grim.

We also came into contact with Ryan, a young man in the Air Force. Ryan was given the smallpox vaccination and had a bad reaction about 10 days later. They found him in his barracks, lethargic, staggering, slurring his words, with apparent memory loss. At first they suspected illegal drug use, but after several tests, diagnosed him with ADEM. Like Joe, he was comatose and on a respirator for a time and was also treated with IVIG. To my knowledge, there have only been two young men who have gotten ADEM from the smallpox vaccination since Joe came down with it. We still hear from Justin & Ryan and their families from time to time, and other families too.

As time goes on, more and more people are calling me to talk about their son's reactions to their military vaccinations. So far, only two have been diagnosed with ADEM, but others have experienced different adverse reactions to either the smallpox vaccination or to a "cocktail" of vaccinations. Some of our recruits are given 6 or 8 vaccinations in one day, making it impossible for the doctors to know which one has caused the problems. Some reactions are mild but many are severe, life changing and even life threatening. I wonder why these fine young men aren't given their vaccinations one or two at a time, so the doctors will be able to treat adverse reactions more easily — and be more able to determine which one caused the problem.

Last spring, Joe returned to Bethesda Naval Medical Center — the same hospital where he was treated when he first came back to America. He lived across the street in Mercy Hall, the barracks for the Wounded Warrior Program, for five months. The rooms there are all handicap accessible to meet the needs of multiple injuries. He went there for his medical board evaluations but also had a lively social life. They take the Wounded Warriors to lots of social events — dinners, professional sports, tours, special events, etc. — and he had the opportunity to meet professional athletes, performers, politicians, beauty queens, retired Marines, the list goes on and on — even to the President of the United States. People want to shake his hand, they want to thank him for his service, for putting his life on the line for them. It's done a lot for his self esteem.

Medically, Joe continues to deal with multiple problems. But there are also successes. He takes prescriptions which help him to walk, but has knee problems. He still has bladder problems but with proper medication, he is able to deal with it. He has some short term memory problems and the medications he takes make him drowsy, but he is able to drive a car during the non-drowsy times. He walks short distances and no longer uses a wheelchair.

Since the first phone call on that first day, the military system has worked for him. Even though there have been a few glitches, we have been able to navigate our way. We had some major problems with Tri-Care but eventually, all medical needs were addressed, and every request we made was honored.

Our major disappointment has been with TSGLI, insurance that covers war zone traumatic injuries but has denied coverage of Joe's injury.

Joe's care has been a success story for the different military branches — the Army personnel in Germany, the Air Force personnel on the medivac flights, the Navy personnel at Bethesda, and the many, many Marine Corps personnel. They have all been wonderful, working together and separately to get the job done. They are all my heroes.

There are other heroes in this story — friends, co-workers, neighbors, family, even complete strangers — so many people who have come to our aid and helped us through the past two years. They are all my heroes.

As we look to the future, we know that more heroes will come and go in our lives. We look forward to the challenges that life will send our way. Joe will soon be out of the Marine Corps and will be sent from the embracing arms of the military to the long term care of the Veterans Administration. We hope that it goes well. He has recently gone back to college, part time, but is still undecided on a major. He seems to be leaning toward the science field, possibly even medicine.

Recently, we attended another Marine Parents Conference, this one held in Washington D.C., and enjoyed being with our Marine Parents friends again. We went on a tour to the Marine Corps Museum, saw the Silent Drill Team of 8th & I Battalion, and visited the Iwo Jima Memorial at Arlington Cemetery. It was all so very inspiring. On the second day we got up before dawn, got on a charter bus, and went to the National Mall. There, we watched as one group left to run with Marines from Recruit Station Baltimore. Then, along with 40 or so other Marine parents, I fell into step behind my hero — walking with his cane — as he lead our group on a half mile walk. We weren't the smartest looking group, and we did a pitiful job in our warm-up exercises — with looks of horror on our faces when the word "push-ups" came out of our "drill instructor's" mouth! Yes, we were a pathetic looking bunch, but we all fell in and did our best as each parent's mind wandered to thoughts of their own heroes — their own children, all at various stages of their Marine Corps lives. We were pitiful looking, but proud, and we walked smartly behind Joe — the representative for each of their children — and we were one. These parents, and all military parents, they are my heroes.

Joe rode his hand cycle in the 2008 Marine Corps Marathon, and I ran the 10K again. This time he rode for Achilles Track Club and we were excited to meet the other members of the team, handicapped for various reasons but participating as the true athletes that they are. They are my heroes.

I have met many former military, both men and women. People who wanted to shake my hand. People who wanted to give me a hug. People who wanted to thank me for raising a child such as Joe. People who wanted to thank me for my sacrifice. I am always in awe of these people. The ones who have served their country and sacrificed for their country. They are my heroes.

I suppose I have many heroes, and I will forever be inspired by them, and grateful to them. They are the backbone of this great country.

To each of you who has taken the time to read this book, I send a big Oo-rah and Semper Fi. Let it inspire your life as it has inspired mine. Semper Fi, the creed of the Marine Corps, Always Faithful. Thank a Marine, soldier, airman or sailor today — make them your heroes too.

Acknowledgments

First and foremost, I would like to thank my son, Josef, for allowing me to tell his story and reveal even the most intimate details of his treatment. Without him, there would be no story to tell.

I also thank my other son, Steven, for being there, every step of the way, for this amazing journey. He put his life on hold and in the course of two short months, accompanied me to Germany then to Bethesda; made a second trip to Bethesda, and a third trip to Springfield. He would have made a fourth trip, but was stopped by a snow storm.

To my late husband, Lou, who held it together as best he could but succumbed to the ravages of his diseases: Alzheimer's Disease and heart disease.

To my sisters, Teri and Sheri, who did what they could to help Lou while I was away. Especially Teri and her children, who took him in and treated him like a member of their family.

To Dr. Montgomery and everyone at the Vaccine Health Center, who continue to advocate for Joe and monitor his health. The dozens of doctors, nurses, therapists, corpsmen, and other medical personnel who worked with Joe during his recovery. The pilots and crew of the medivac planes that brought him home. The non-medical personnel who visited him in the hospital — chaplains, social workers, volunteers, etc.

I thank the other patients and their families, who have shared their stories and become so important in our lives.

I thank those proud Marines of the 1/24 who served with Joe in Iraq and kept such close tabs on him during his recovery. Also the Marines of the 3/24, who have taken such good care of him since his return to Springfield. A big "oo-rah" goes out to them!

I thank the staff at St. John's Medical Center in Springfield, Missouri, including the physical therapy and pool therapy staff. Again, the other patients who meant so much to his recovery.

I thank our neighbors and friends, who cared for us and supported us, going way beyond what they had to do to help us.

I thank our friends from Marine Parents, A Heart of a Marine, Achilles Track Club, Semper Fi Fund, and all the other organizations that helped us.

Last, but certainly not least, I thank my dad and step-mother, Carlyle and Grace Lucas, who were there every step of the way. Taking care of the house, visiting Lou in the nursing home and hospital, traveling into town numerous times to make sure Joe and I were doing well.

So many people have given so much, we are eternally grateful, and truly humbled. To each and every one, a heartfelt "thank you, and God bless".

LaVergne, TN USA
26 October 2009

161907LV00002BA/2/P